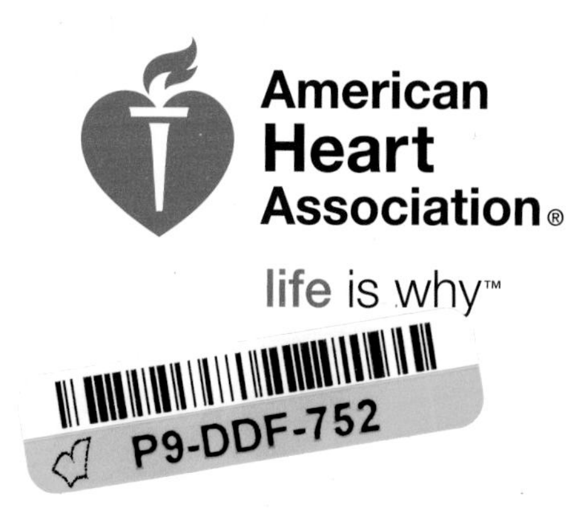

Heartsaver® FIRST AID CPR AED

STUDENT WORKBOOK

ISBN 978-1-61669-424-1
Printed in the United States of America
First American Heart Association Printing April 2016
10 9 8 7

Acknowledgments

The American Heart Association thanks the following people for their contributions to the development of this workbook: Jeff A. Woodin, NREMT-P; Mary Fran Hazinski, RN, MSN; Robert Lee Hanna; Kostas Alibertis, CCEMT-P; Tony Connelly, EMT-P, BHSc, PGCEd; Brian E. Grunau, MD; Jeanette Previdi, MPH, BSN, RN-BC; Mark Terry, MPA, NREMT-P; Moira Muldoon; Brenda Schoolfield; and the AHA Heartsaver Project Team.

To find out about any updates or corrections to this text, visit **www.heart.org/cpr**, navigate to the page for this course, and click on "Updates."

Contents

CONTENTS

life is why.™

At the American Heart Association, we want people to experience more of life's precious moments. That's why we've made better heart and brain health our mission. It's also why we remain committed to exceptional training–the act of bringing resuscitation science to life–through genuine partnership with you. Only through our continued collaboration and dedication can we truly make a difference and save lives.

Until there's a world free of heart disease and stroke, the American Heart Association will be there, working with you to make a healthier, longer life possible for everyone.

Why do we do what we do? life is why.

Life Is Why is a celebration of life. A simple yet powerful answer to the question of why we should all be healthy in heart and mind. It also explains why we do what we do: Lifesaving work. Every day.

Throughout your student manual, you will find information that correlates what you are learning in this class to **Life Is Why** and the importance of cardiovascular care. Look for the **Life Is Why** icon (shown at right), and remember that what you are learning today has an impact on the mission of the American Heart Association.

We encourage you to discover your **Why** and share it with others. Ask yourself, what are the moments, people, and experiences I live for? What brings me joy, wonder, and happiness? Why am I partnering with the AHA to help save lives? Why is cardiovascular care important to me? The answer to these questions is your **Why.**

Instructions

Please find on the back of this page a chance for you to participate in the AHA's mission and **Life Is Why** campaign. Complete this activity by filling in the blank with the word that describes your **Why.**

Share your **"_______ Is Why"** with the people you love, and ask them to discover their **Why.**

Talk about it. Share it. Post it. Live it. #lifeiswhy #CPRSavesLives

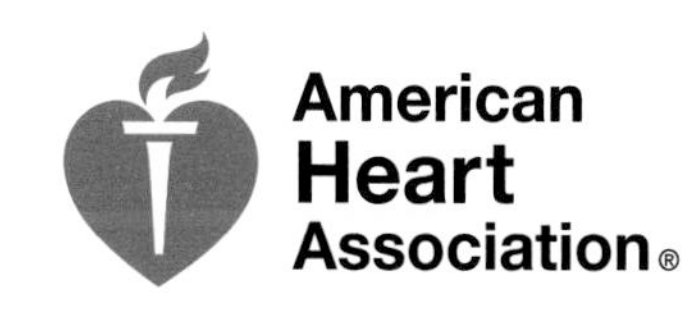

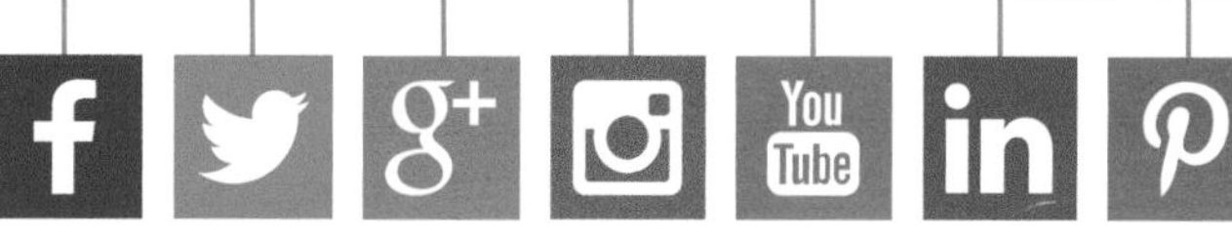

_______________ is why.

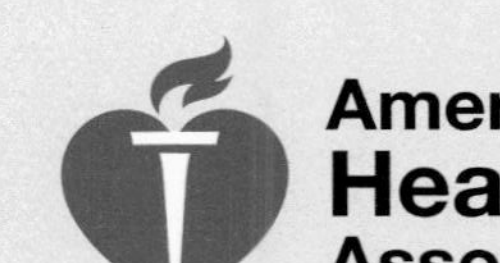

Introduction

Heartsaver First Aid CPR AED Course

Welcome to the Heartsaver First Aid CPR AED Course. During this course, you will gain knowledge and skills that may help save a life.

In this course, you will learn the basics of first aid, the most common life-threatening emergencies, how to recognize them, and how to help. You will also learn how to recognize when someone needs CPR, how to call for help, and how give CPR and use an AED.

What You Will Learn in This Course

The most important goal of this course is to teach you to act in an emergency. Sometimes, people don't act because they are afraid of doing the wrong thing. Recognizing that something is wrong and getting help on the way by phoning 9-1-1 are the most important things you can do.

Once you phone 9-1-1, the dispatcher—the person who answers 9-1-1 calls—will guide you in what to do until help arrives. People with advanced training (emergency medical technicians, paramedics, and others) usually arrive and take over soon after you call. Your job is to recognize when something is wrong, get help on the way if it's needed, and give first aid care or CPR until someone with more advanced training arrives and takes over. In this course, we'll also cover the Good Samaritan laws, which protect CPR rescuers.

Life Is Why

Life Is Why

At the American Heart Association, we want people to experience more of life's precious moments. What you learn in this course can help build healthier, longer lives for everyone.

Heartsaver First Aid CPR AED Knowledge and Skills

Your Student Workbook contains all of the information that you need to be able to understand and perform lifesaving and first aid skills correctly. During the course, you will be given the opportunity to practice these skills and receive valuable coaching from your instructor.

The video in the course will cover many, but not all, of the skills discussed in this workbook. So, it is important to study your workbook to be fully prepared to help in an emergency.

Successful Course Completion

During the course, you will be asked to practice and demonstrate important skills. As you read and study this workbook, pay particular attention to these skills.

If you complete all course requirements and demonstrate the skills correctly, you'll receive a course completion card.

How to Use the Student Workbook

Take time to read and study the Student Workbook carefully. You should use this workbook before, during, and after the course.

Before the course	• Read and study the workbook. • Look at the step-by-step instructions, skills summaries, and pictures. • Take notes. • Make a list of questions to ask your instructor.
During the course	• Refer to the workbook during the video demonstrations and hands-on practice.
After the course	• Review the step-by-step instructions, skills summaries, and pictures. • Keep your workbook readily available for reference during emergencies.

How Often Training Is Needed

Review your Student Workbook and Quick Reference Guide often to recall important skills. Your course completion card is valid for 2 years.

First Aid Course Objectives

This course includes both First Aid and CPR AED. At the end of the First Aid portion, you will be able to

- List the priorities, roles, and responsibilities of first aid rescuers
- Describe the key steps in first aid
- Remove protective gloves (skill you will demonstrate)
- Find the problem (skill you will demonstrate)
- Describe the assessment and first aid actions for the following life-threatening conditions: heart attack, difficulty breathing, choking, severe bleeding, shock, and stroke
- Describe when and how to help a choking adult or child
- Demonstrate how to help a choking infant
- Use an epinephrine pen (skill you will demonstrate)
- Control bleeding and bandaging (skill you will demonstrate)
- Recognize elements of common injuries

- Recognize elements of common illnesses
- Describe how to find information on preventing illness and injury
- Recognize the legal questions that apply to first aid rescuers

See the CPR AED section of this workbook for the CPR AED course objectives.

Heartsaver First Aid CPR AED Terms and Concepts

What You Will Learn

In this section, you will learn key terms and concepts that are used throughout the Heartsaver Course. They are the foundation for understanding the material presented in this workbook.

First Aid

First aid is the immediate care that you give a person with an illness or injury before rescuers with more advanced training arrive and take over.

First aid may be started by anyone in any situation. It may help an ill or injured person recover more completely or more quickly. In serious emergencies, first aid can mean the difference between life and death.

Most of the time, you'll give first aid for minor illnesses or injuries. But you may also give first aid for problems that could become life threatening, such as providing aid for a heart attack, bandaging for severe bleeding, or giving epinephrine for a severe allergic reaction.

In this course, you will learn and practice first aid skills, which will help you remember what to do in a real emergency.

Responsive vs Unresponsive

You should know that during an emergency, it's possible that someone might become unresponsive. Here is how to decide if someone is responsive or unresponsive:

- *Responsive:* Someone who is responsive will move, speak, blink, or otherwise react to you when you tap him and ask if he's OK.
- *Unresponsive:* Someone who does not move, speak, blink, or otherwise react is unresponsive.

If someone is unresponsive, you will learn to check to see if the person needs CPR.

Agonal Gasps

A person in cardiac arrest will not be breathing normally or only gasping. When we refer to *gasps*, we mean agonal gasps. Agonal gasps are frequently present in the first minutes after sudden cardiac arrest.

If a person is gasping, it usually looks like he is drawing air in very quickly. He may open his mouth and move his jaw, head, or neck.

The gasp may sound like a snort, snore, or groan. These gasps may appear forceful or weak. Some time may pass between gasps because they often happen at a slow rate.

Gasping is not regular or normal breathing. It's a sign of cardiac arrest in someone who is unresponsive.

Cardiopulmonary Resuscitation (CPR)

CPR stands for cardiopulmonary resuscitation. When a person's heart stops suddenly, providing CPR can double or even triple the chances of survival.

CPR is made up of 2 skills:

- Providing compressions
- Giving breaths

A compression is the act of pushing hard and fast on the chest. When you push on the chest, you pump blood to the brain and heart. To give CPR, you provide sets of 30 compressions and 2 breaths.

See the "CPR and AED" part of this workbook for more information.

Automated External Defibrillator (AED)

AED stands for automated external defibrillator. It's a lightweight, portable device that can detect an abnormal cardiac rhythm requiring treatment with a shock. An AED can deliver a shock to convert the rhythm back to normal.

When you give first aid, you will need to get the first aid kit and sometimes an AED. AEDs should be located in a company's main office, a building's high-traffic area, a break room, or a high-risk area, such as a gym—anywhere the most people will see and have access to them when an emergency occurs.

It is very important that you become aware of the location of the nearest first aid kit and AED so that you may provide the best possible help to someone who is ill or injured.

Adults, Children, and Infants

This workbook presents specific Heartsaver skills and actions for helping an ill or injured adult, child, or infant until the next level of care arrives. For the purposes of this course, we use the following age definitions:

Adult	Adolescent (after the onset of puberty) and older
Child	1 year of age to puberty
Infant	Less than 1 year of age

Signs of puberty include chest or underarm hair in males and any breast development in females.

Treat anyone who has signs of puberty as an adult. If you are in doubt about whether someone is an adult or a child, provide emergency care as if the person is an adult.

Phone 9-1-1

In this course, we say "phone 9-1-1." You may have a different emergency response number. If you do, phone your emergency response number instead of 9-1-1.

In an emergency, use the most readily available phone to phone 9-1-1. This may be your cell phone or the cell phone of someone who comes to help. In some cases, you may need to use another type of phone. After calling 9-1-1, make sure the phone is on speaker mode, if possible, so that the person providing emergency care can talk to the dispatcher.

Part 1: First Aid Basics

Topics Covered

Topics covered in this part are

- Duties, roles, and responsibilities of the first aid rescuer
- Steps of first aid

As you read and study this part, pay particular attention to these 2 skills that you will be asked to demonstrate during the course:

- Removing protective gloves
- Finding the problem

Duties, Roles, and Responsibilities of First Aid Rescuers

Some people may be required to perform first aid while working. For example, law enforcement officers, firefighters, flight attendants, lifeguards, and park rangers may have a duty to give first aid when they are working. When off duty, they can choose whether or not to provide first aid.

It's important for you to know that you may learn private things about the person you are helping. Keep private information private. Share information about an ill or injured person only with emergency responders when they take over.

Your Role in the EMS System

Your role as a first aid rescuer is to

- Recognize that an emergency exists
- Make sure the scene is safe for you and the ill or injured person
- Phone 9-1-1
- Provide care until someone with more advanced training arrives and takes over

When you phone 9-1-1, you activate the network of emergency responders, or emergency medical services (EMS). Getting help on the way quickly in an emergency can save a life.

Deciding to Provide First Aid

Providing first aid may be part of your job description. If so, you must help while you're working. However, when you're off duty, you can choose whether or not to provide first aid.

Asking to Give First Aid

When you come upon an ill or injured person and the person responds, introduce yourself as a first aid provider before you touch the person. Ask if you may help. Anyone has the right to refuse.

Asking to Give First Aid
☐ When you come upon an ill or injured person and the person responds, introduce yourself as a first aid provider before you touch the person.
☐ Ask if you may help. • If the person agrees, give first aid. • If the person refuses, phone 9-1-1 and stay with him until help arrives. • If the person is confused or can't answer, assume the person wants help.

Maintaining the First Aid Kit

One of the responsibilities of a first aid provider is to maintain the first aid kit. It's important that the first aid kit contain the supplies you'll need for most common emergencies.

See "Part 6: First Aid Resources" for a list of what is usually kept in a kit. Your kit may be different, however, so please check the first aid kit against the list to see if there are additional items you need to add. Be sure to restock it after any emergency.

Maintaining the First Aid Kit
☐ Keep the supplies in a sturdy, watertight container that is clearly labeled.
☐ Know where the first aid kit is.
☐ Replace what you use so that the kit will be ready for the next emergency.
☐ Check the kit at the beginning of each work period for expired supplies and to make sure it is complete and ready for an emergency.

Good Samaritan Laws

If you have questions about whether or not it's legal to provide someone first aid, you should know that all states have Good Samaritan laws. These laws protect anyone who provides first aid. They differ from state to state, so be sure to check the laws in your area.

Key Steps of First Aid

For every emergency, follow the key steps of first aid:

- Assess the scene.
- Phone for help.
- Take universal precautions.
- Find the problem.
- Protect the person's privacy.

Assess the Scene

First, make sure the scene is safe. Be aware of any danger for you, the ill or injured person, and anyone else nearby.

This is an important step. Do it every time you are providing help. Continue to assess the scene while you provide first aid to be aware of anything that might change and make it unsafe. You can't help anyone if you're injured yourself.

The first step in any first aid action is to make sure the scene is safe.

Questions for Assessing the Scene

When you look around, ask yourself these questions:

	Question	Explanation
Danger	Is there danger for you or the ill or injured person?	Move an injured person only if he is in danger or if you need to move him to safely provide first aid or CPR.
Help	Are others around to help?	If so, have someone phone 9-1-1. If no one else is near, phone for help yourself.
Who	Who is ill or injured?	Can you tell how many people are hurt and what happened?
Where	Where are you?	You'll need to tell others how to get to you—in particular, the 9-1-1 dispatcher. If there are other bystanders at the scene, send one of them to meet the emergency responders and lead them to the scene.

As you assess the need for first aid, it's important to know when and how to phone for help. Phoning 9-1-1 activates the EMS network of responders.

Make sure you know the nearest location of a phone to use in an emergency (Figure 1). Often, the first aid kit and AED are stored at the same location as the emergency phone.

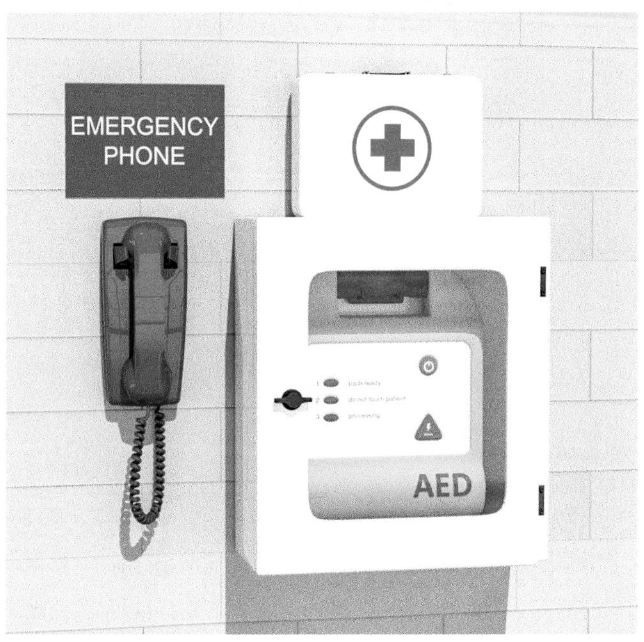

Figure 1. Know the location of the nearest phone to use in an emergency. You also should know where the first aid kit and AED are stored.

When to Phone for Help

Your company may have some instructions about when you should phone the emergency response number (or 9-1-1).

As a general rule, you should phone 9-1-1 and ask for help whenever someone is seriously ill or injured or you are not sure what to do in an emergency.

Some examples of when you should phone 9-1-1 are if the ill or injured person

- Doesn't respond to voice or touch
- Has chest discomfort, signaling possible heart attack
- Has signs of a stroke
- Has a problem breathing
- Has a severe injury or burn
- Has severe bleeding
- Has a seizure
- Suddenly can't move a part of the body
- Has received an electric shock
- Has been exposed to poison

You will learn more about the signs and first aid actions for these medical and injury emergencies later in this workbook.

How to Phone for Help

It's also important for you to know how to phone for help from your location. Do you know how to activate the emergency response number in your workplace? For example, is it necessary to dial 9 for an outside line, or is there an internal number to phone that will notify responders who are on-site?

For the purposes of this course, we will say "phone 9-1-1" as the emergency response number.

Write the emergency response number on your Quick Reference Guide, in the first aid kit, and near the telephone. You should also write it here.

Write your emergency response number here:

____

Who Should Phone for Help

If other people are available, you can ask someone else to phone 9-1-1 and get the first aid kit and AED. If you are alone and have a cell phone, call 9-1-1 and put the phone on speaker mode so that you can follow the dispatcher's instructions. Here is a summary:

If you are	Then you should
Alone	☐ Shout for help. ☐ If no one answers and the person needs immediate care and you have a cell phone, phone 9-1-1 and put the phone on speaker mode. ☐ The dispatcher will provide further instruction, such as how to give first aid, give CPR, or use an AED.
With others	☐ Stay with the ill or injured person and be prepared to give first aid or CPR if you know how. ☐ Send someone else to phone 9-1-1 and get the first aid kit and AED if available. ☐ Have the person put the phone on speaker mode so that you can receive further instruction from the dispatcher.

Follow the Dispatcher's Instructions

When you're on the phone with the dispatcher, don't hang up until the dispatcher tells you to. Answering the dispatcher's questions won't delay arrival of help. Always be aware of your surroundings—knowing the address of your location will help emergency responders reach you more quickly.

Take Universal Precautions

Once you have assessed scene safety, there are universal precautions you should take. These precautions are called *universal* because you should treat all blood and other body fluids as if they contain germs that can cause diseases.

Personal Protective Equipment

Your first aid kit includes personal protective equipment (PPE), such as eye protection and medical gloves. While you are giving first aid, these help keep you safe from blood and body fluids, such as saliva and urine. The first aid kit also contains a mask for giving breaths in case you need to give CPR.

Because some people are allergic to latex or have developed sensitivity to latex that can cause serious reactions, you should use nonlatex gloves if at all possible.

Actions for Universal Precautions

Take the following actions to protect yourself from disease and injury:

Actions for Universal Precautions
☐ Wear PPE whenever necessary (Figure 2). • Wear protective gloves whenever you give first aid. • Wear eye protection if the ill or injured person is bleeding.
☐ Place all disposable equipment that has touched blood or body fluids containing blood in a biohazard waste bag (Figure 3) or as required by your workplace.
☐ To dispose of the biohazard waste bag, follow your company's plan for disposing of hazardous waste.
☐ After properly removing your gloves, wash your hands well with soap and lots of water for 20 seconds.

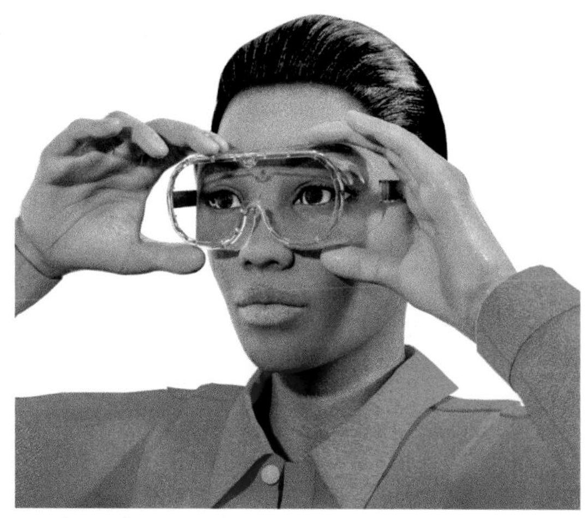

Figure 2. Wear protective gloves whenever you give first aid, and wear eye protection if the ill or injured person is bleeding.

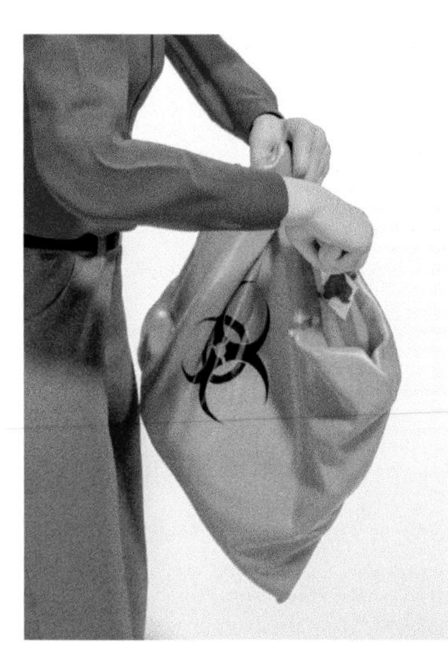

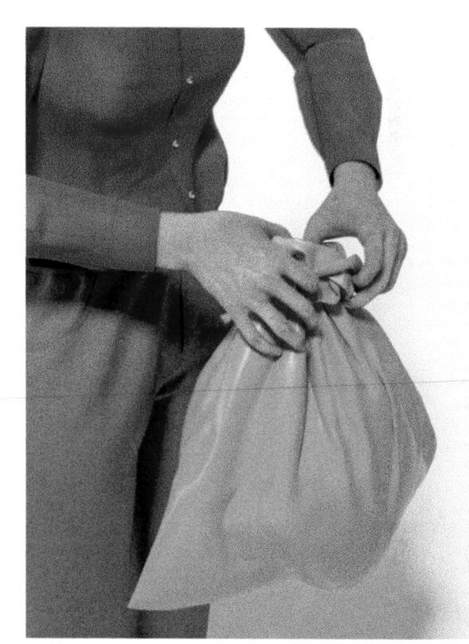

Figure 3. Place all disposable equipment that has touched body fluids, including the gloves you wore, in a biohazard waste bag if one is available. Dispose of the bag according to company policy.

Actions for Exposure to Blood

You should always wear PPE whenever possible. However, if the person's blood does make contact with your skin, or splashes in your eyes or mouth, take these steps:

Actions for Exposure to Blood
☐ Remove your gloves if you are wearing them.
☐ Immediately wash your hands and rinse the contact area with soap and lots of water for 20 seconds.
☐ Rinse your eyes, your nose, or the inside of your mouth with plenty of water if body fluids splattered in any of these areas.
☐ Contact a healthcare provider as soon as possible.

Remove Protective Gloves Properly

Because of the risk of infection, using protective gloves and taking them off correctly are important steps when it comes to your safety and the safety of others.

Always dispose of protective gloves properly so that anyone else who comes in contact with the biohazard waste bag does not get exposed to blood or body fluids.

Actions for Removing Protective Gloves

Here is the correct way to remove protective gloves (Figure 4):

Actions for Removing Protective Gloves
☐ Grip one glove on the outside near the cuff, and peel it down until it comes off inside out (Figure 4A).
☐ Cup it with your other gloved hand (Figure 4B).
☐ Place 2 fingers of your bare hand inside the cuff of the glove that is still on your other hand (Figure 4C).
☐ Peel that glove off so that it comes off inside out with the first glove inside it (Figure 4D).
☐ If blood or blood-containing material is on the gloves, dispose of the gloves properly. • Put the gloves in a biohazard waste bag. • If you do not have a biohazard waste bag, put the gloves in a plastic bag that can be sealed before you dispose of it.
☐ Wash your hands well. You should always wash your hands after removing gloves, just in case some blood or body fluids came in contact with your hands.

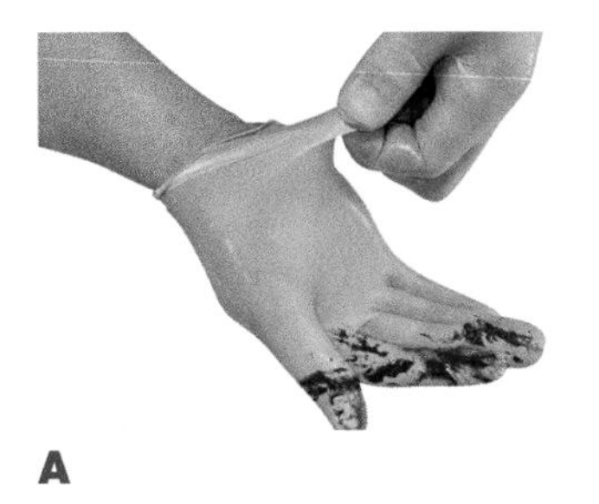
A

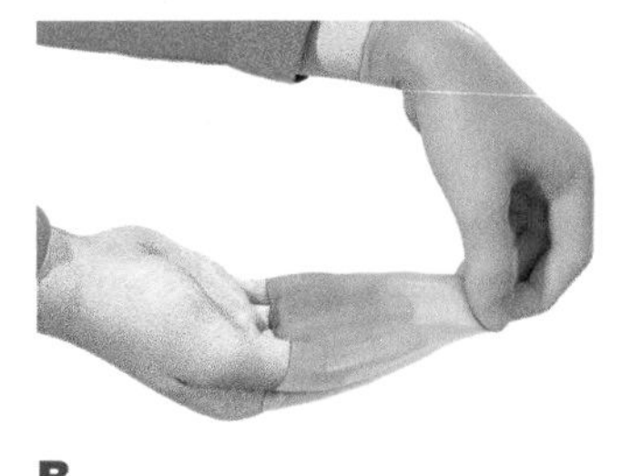
B

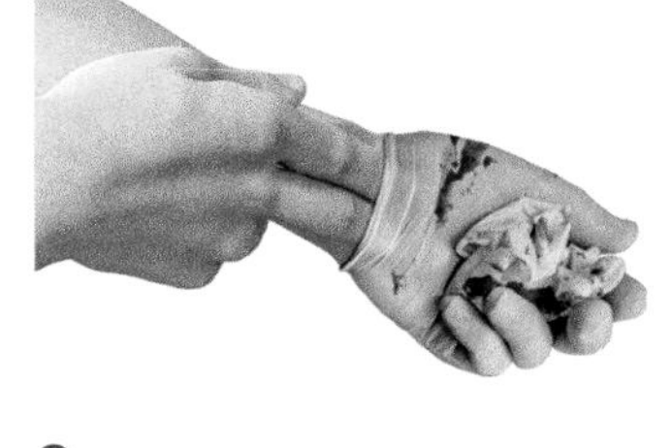
C

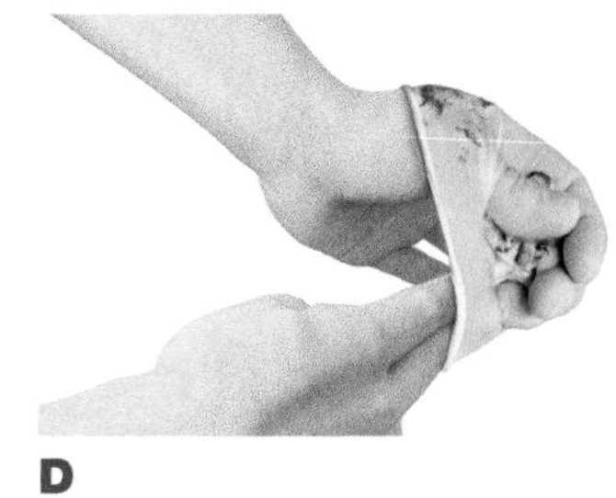
D

Figure 4. Proper removal of protective gloves without touching the outside of the gloves.

Practice Good Hand Hygiene

Even if you've been wearing protective gloves, you should always wash your hands just in case some blood or body fluids came in contact with your hands. Also, good hand hygiene helps prevent the spread of germs. Washing your hands well is one of the most important protections you have against infection.

Actions for Washing Hands Well

Actions for Washing Hands Well
☐ Wet your hands with clean running water (warm if available) and apply soap.
☐ Rub hands together and scrub all surfaces of hands and fingers over for at least 20 seconds (Figure 5).
☐ Rinse hands with lots of running water.
☐ Dry your hands using a paper towel or air dryer. If possible, use your paper towel to turn off the faucet.

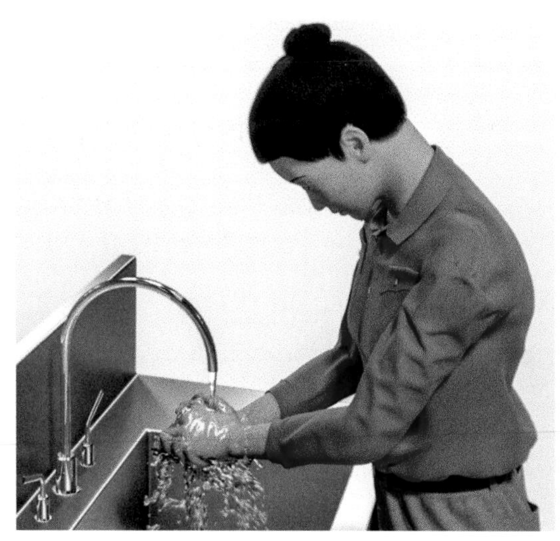

Figure 5. Wash your hands well with soap and lots of water after taking off your gloves.

Using Waterless Hand Sanitizer

If you can't wash your hands right away, use waterless hand sanitizer. Rub your hands together so that the sanitizer covers the tops and bottoms of both hands and all fingers. Then, let the sanitizer air dry.

As soon as you can, wash your hands with soap and water.

Find the Problem

Before you give first aid, you must assess the ill or injured person to find out what the problem is.

- Check to see if the person is responsive or unresponsive (Figure 6). If the person is unresponsive, check for breathing.
- If the person is breathing and doesn't need immediate first aid, look for any obvious signs of injury, such as bleeding, broken bones, burns, or bites.
- Look for any medical information jewelry (Figure 7). This tells you if the person has a serious medical condition.
- Follow the actions outlined in the "Actions for Finding the Problem" section.

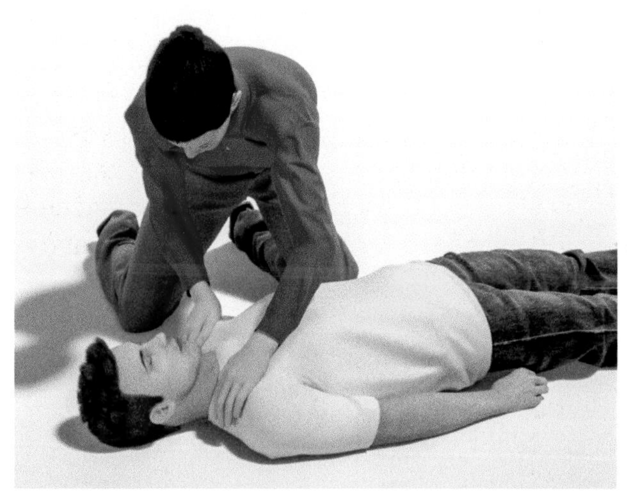

Figure 6. Check to see if the person is responsive or unresponsive. Tap and shout, "Are you OK?"

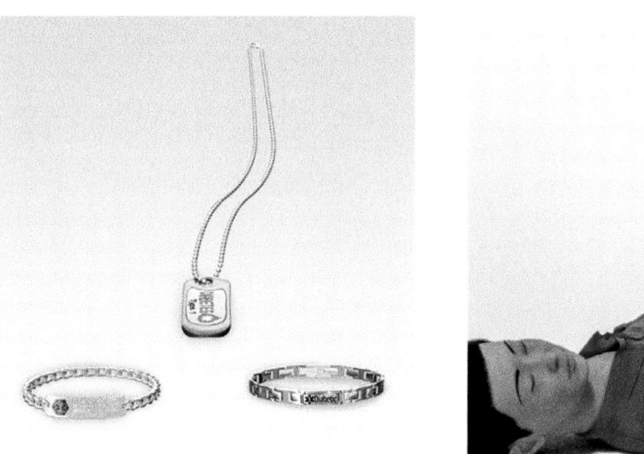

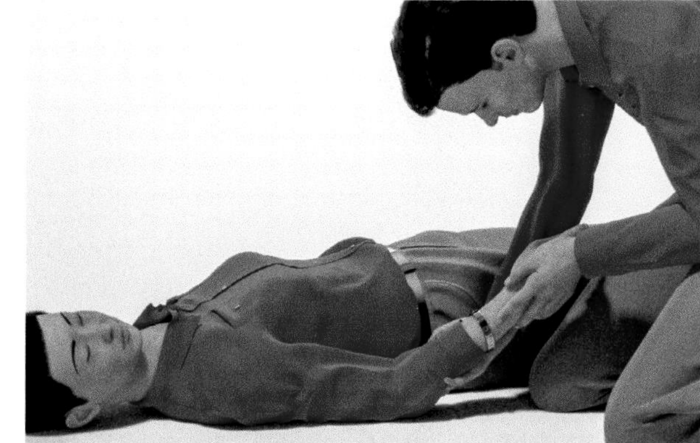

Figure 7. Look for medical information jewelry.

Actions for Finding the Problem

The following steps will help you find out what the problem is. They are listed in order of importance, with the most important step listed first.

Actions for Finding the Problem
☐ Make sure the scene is safe.
☐ Check to see if the person responds. Approach the person, tap him, and shout, "Are you OK? Are you OK?"

If the person is *responsive*	If the person is *unresponsive*
☐ Ask what the problem is.	☐ Shout for help and phone 9-1-1. • Phone or send someone to phone 9-1-1 and get a first aid kit and AED. • If you are alone and have a cell phone, put it on speaker mode and phone 9-1-1. Go get the first aid kit and AED yourself.

(continued)

(continued)

If the person is ***responsive***	If the person is ***unresponsive***
☐ If the person only moves, moans, or groans, shout for help. Phone or send someone to phone 9-1-1 and get the first aid kit and AED.	☐ Check for breathing. • If the person is breathing normally, stay with him until advanced help arrives. Check for injuries and medical information jewelry. • If the person is not breathing normally or only gasping, begin CPR and use an AED. See the "CPR and AED" part of this workbook.
☐ Check for breathing. • If the person is breathing and doesn't need immediate first aid, look for any obvious signs of injury, such as bleeding, broken bones, burns, or bites. • Look for any medical information jewelry. This tells you if the person has a serious medical condition.	☐ Stay with the person until advanced help arrives.

Use Caution When Moving an Ill or Injured Person

When giving first aid, you might wonder, "Should I move an ill or injured person?"

The answer is generally no. This is especially important if you suspect that the person may have a pelvic or spinal injury.

However, there are times when the person should be moved, such as the following:

- If the area is unsafe for you or the ill or injured person, move to a safe location.
- If a person is unresponsive and breathing normally, you may roll the person onto his side. By rolling the person onto his side, you may help keep his airway open in case he vomits.

One way to move someone is to drag the person by his clothes (Figure 8). Place your hands on the person's shoulders, grab his clothes, and pull him to safety.

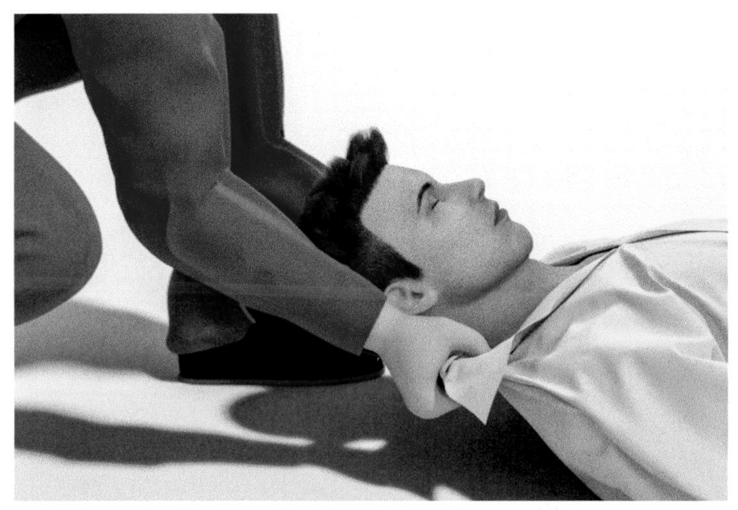

Figure 8. The shoulder pull is a way to move an ill or injured person.

Protect the Person's Privacy

As a first aid rescuer, you may learn private things about the people you help, such as their medical conditions. Give all information about an ill or injured person to EMS rescuers. If you are in your workplace, also give this information to your company's emergency response program supervisor. You may need to fill out a report for your company.

If an emergency does happen in your workplace, you must not share this information with other coworkers. Keep private things private.

First Aid Basics: Review Questions

Question	Your Notes
1. When you are providing first aid, you should a. Wear PPE b. Only wear PPE if the person is someone you do not know c. Not be concerned about PPE if you wash your hands d. Use cloth gloves to protect your hands	
2. When you phone for help, you should stay on the line with the dispatcher until a. People with more advanced training arrive b. The dispatcher tells you it's OK to hang up	

(continued)

(continued)

Question	Your Notes
3. After giving first aid at your workplace, you a. Can talk about what happened with anyone you want b. Cannot discuss anything with coworkers; you must keep private things private c. Can speak to a reporter about the incident d. Can discuss the incident with your immediate coworkers only	
4. You should wash your hands for at least a. 10 seconds b. 15 seconds c. 20 seconds d. 3 minutes	
5. When assessing the scene, you should consider which of the following *(circle all that apply)*: a. Danger to yourself and others b. How many people are injured or ill c. Where the location is d. Where the nearest telephone is	
6. You should replace any supplies you use from the first aid kit. True False	

Answers: **1.** a, **2.** b, **3.** b, **4.** c, **5.** All, **6.** True

Part 2: Medical Emergencies

Some conditions are life threatening. Acting quickly can help someone stay alive.

At the most basic level, people need to breathe and keep blood pumping inside their bodies. With a little bit of knowledge, first aid rescuers often can help people do just that.

In this part, we look at first aid actions for medical emergencies, including breathing problems, severe choking, heart attack, and stroke.

Your actions in the first few minutes when you see the signs of any of these conditions could help save a life!

Topics Covered

Topics covered in this part are

- Breathing problems
- Choking
- Allergic reactions
- Heart attack
- Fainting
- Diabetes and low blood sugar
- Stroke
- Seizure

As you read and study this part, pay particular attention to this skill that you will be asked to demonstrate during the course:

- Using an epinephrine pen

Breathing Problems

Someone may develop mild or severe blockage of the air passages. Someone having a heart attack, having a stroke, or experiencing certain injuries also may have breathing problems.

Asthma

Asthma is a disease of the air passages. A person who is having an asthma attack will have trouble breathing.

Signs of Breathing Problems

You can tell if someone is having trouble breathing if the person

- Is breathing very fast or very slowly
- Is having trouble with every breath
- Has noisy breathing—you hear a sound or whistle as the air enters or leaves the lungs
- Can only make sounds or speak no more than a few words at a time in between breaths although the person is trying to say more

Someone with a medical condition involving breathing problems, such as asthma, usually knows about the condition and what to do. He often carries inhaler medicine, which can help him breathe more easily within minutes of using it.

At times, the person can have such a hard time breathing that he needs help using his inhaler. For this reason, you should be ready to assemble the inhaler and help him use it.

Assemble and Use an Inhaler

Inhalers are made up of 2 parts: the medicine canister and the mouthpiece. A spacer can be attached that makes it easier for the person with the breathing problem to inhale all the medicine (Figure 9).

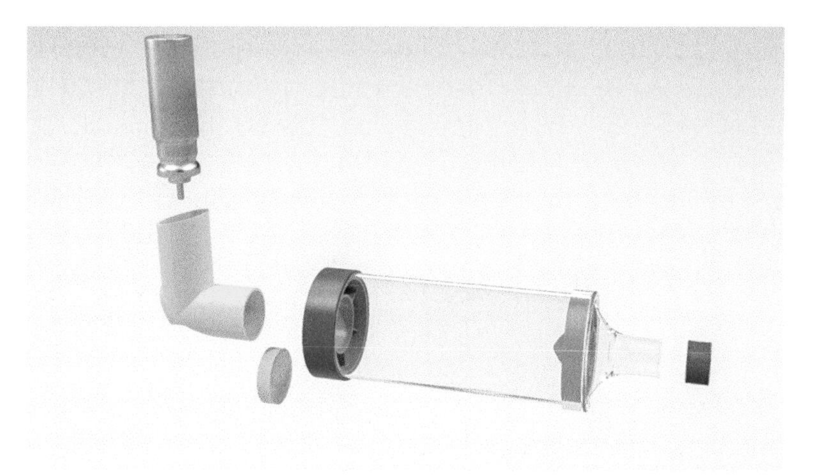

Figure 9. Parts of an inhaler are the medicine canister, mouthpiece, and spacer.

Actions for Assembling and Using an Inhaler

Follow these steps to assemble and use an inhaler:

Actions for Assembling and Using an Inhaler
To assemble the inhaler:
☐ First, shake the medicine.
☐ Put the medicine canister into the mouthpiece.
☐ Remove the cap from the mouthpiece.
☐ Attach a spacer if there is one available and if you know how.
To help someone use an inhaler, ask him to do the following:
☐ Tilt his head back slightly and breathe out slowly.
☐ Place the inhaler or spacer in his mouth (Figure 10).
☐ Push down on the medicine canister.
☐ Breathe in very deeply and slowly.
☐ Hold his breath for about 10 seconds.
☐ Then, breathe out slowly.

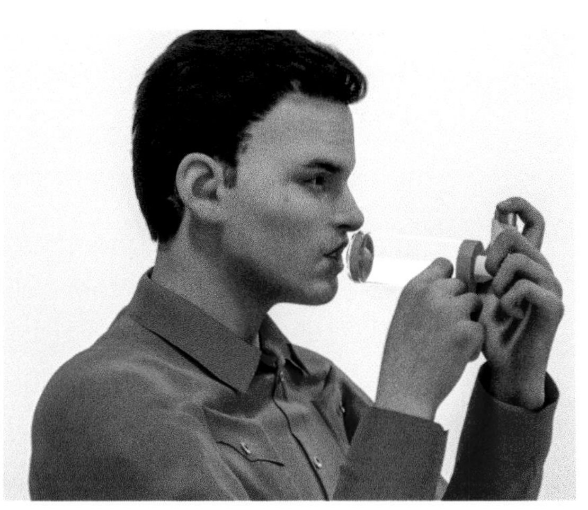

Figure 10. Using an inhaler with a spacer.

Actions for Helping Someone With Breathing Problems

If someone is having breathing problems, follow these first aid action steps to help him:

Actions for Helping Someone With Breathing Problems
☐ Make sure the scene is safe.
☐ Ask the person if he needs help. If he does, ask if he has medicine.
☐ If he has medicine, get it for him. Then, assemble and help him use the inhaler.

(continued)

(continued)

Actions for Helping Someone With Breathing Problems
☐ Phone 9-1-1 if • The person has no medicine • The person does not get better after using his medicine • The person's breathing gets worse • The person has trouble speaking • The person becomes unresponsive
☐ Stay with the person until someone with more advanced training arrives and takes over.

Choking in an Adult, Child, or Infant

What You Will Learn

In this section, you will learn to assess whether someone has a mild or severe block in the airway and how to take action to help.

Overview

Choking is when food or another object gets stuck in the airway in the throat. The object can block the airway and stop air from getting to the lungs.

In adults, choking is often caused by food. In children, choking can be caused by food or another object.

Mild vs Severe Airway Block

Assess Choking and Take Action

The block in the airway that causes choking can be either mild or severe. If the airway block is severe, act quickly. Get the object out so that the person can breathe.

Here is how to assess if someone has a mild or severe airway block and what you should do:

	If Someone	Then Take Action
Mild airway block	• Can talk or make sounds • Can cough loudly	• Stand by and let the person cough. • If you're worried about the person's breathing, phone 9-1-1.
Severe airway block	• Cannot breathe, talk, or make sounds *or* • Has a cough that has no sound *or* • Makes the choking sign	• Act quickly. • Follow the steps to help an adult, child, or infant with a severe airway block.

The Choking Sign

If someone is choking, he might use the choking sign, which is holding the neck with one or both hands (Figure 11).

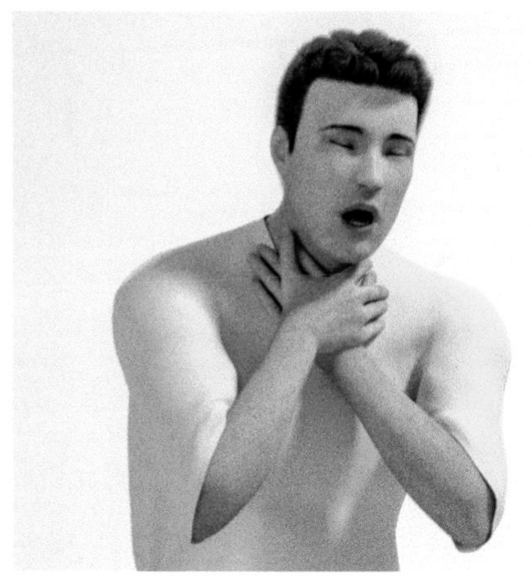
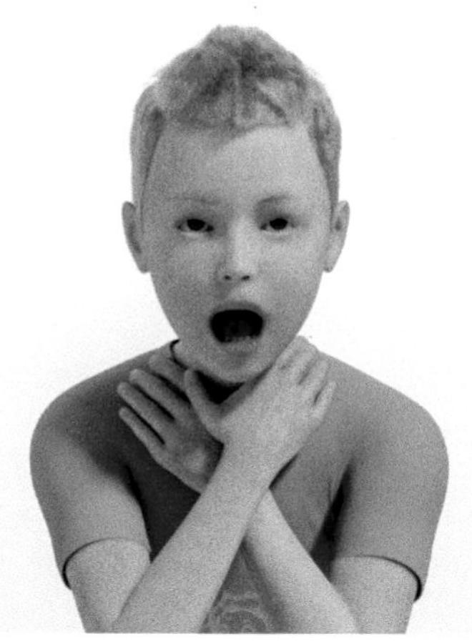

Figure 11. The choking sign: holding the neck with one or both hands.

How to Help an Adult, Child, or Infant Who Has a Severe Airway Block

When an adult or child has a severe airway block, give thrusts slightly above the belly button. These thrusts are called *abdominal thrusts* or the *Heimlich maneuver.* Like a cough, each thrust pushes air from the lungs. This can help move or remove an object that is blocking the airway.

Any person who has received abdominal thrusts for choking should see a healthcare provider as soon as possible.

How to Help a Choking Adult or Child With a Severe Airway Block

Follow these steps to help a choking adult or child who has a severe airway block:

How to Help a Choking Adult or Child With a Severe Airway Block
☐ If you think someone is choking, ask, “Are you choking? Can I help you?”
☐ If the person nods yes, tell him you are going to help.
☐ Stand firmly or kneel behind the person (depending on your size and the size of the person choking). Wrap your arms around the person’s waist so that your fists are in front.
☐ Make a fist with one hand.
☐ Put the thumb side of your fist slightly above the belly button and well below the breastbone.
☐ Grasp the fist with your other hand and give quick upward thrusts into the abdomen (Figure 12).
☐ Give thrusts until the object is forced out and the person can breathe, cough, or speak, or until he becomes unresponsive.

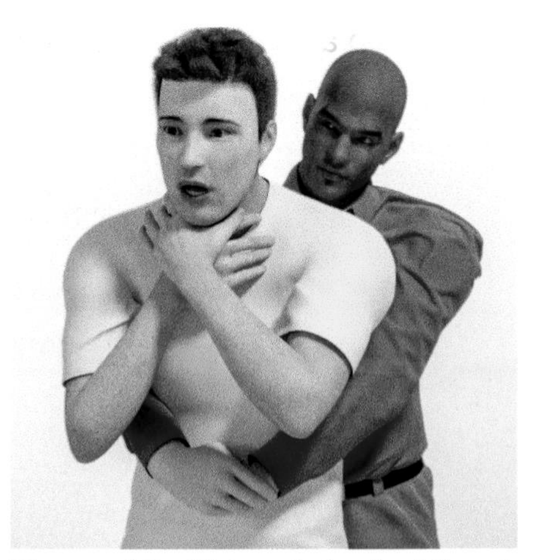

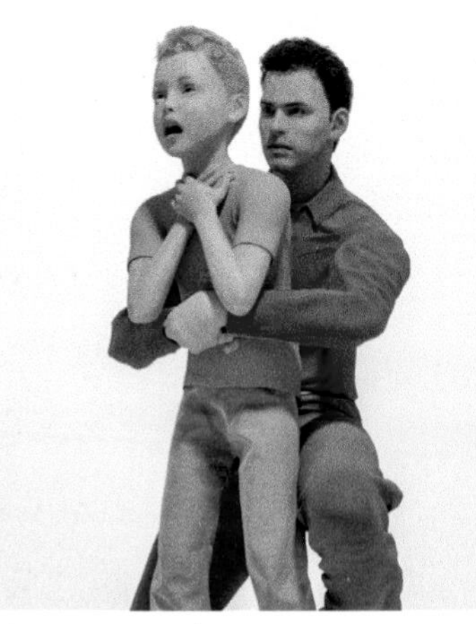

Figure 12. Giving abdominal thrusts (Heimlich maneuver).

How to Help a Choking Pregnant Woman or Large Adult or Child With a Severe Airway Block

If the person who has a severe airway block is pregnant or very large, give chest thrusts instead of abdominal thrusts.

Follow these steps to help a pregnant woman or large adult or child who has a severe airway block:

How to Help a Choking Pregnant Woman or Large Adult or Child With a Severe Airway Block
☐ If you can't wrap your arms fully around the waist, give thrusts on the chest (chest thrusts) instead of on the abdomen.
☐ Put your arms under the armpits and your hands on the lower half of the breastbone.
☐ Pull straight back to give chest thrusts (Figure 13).

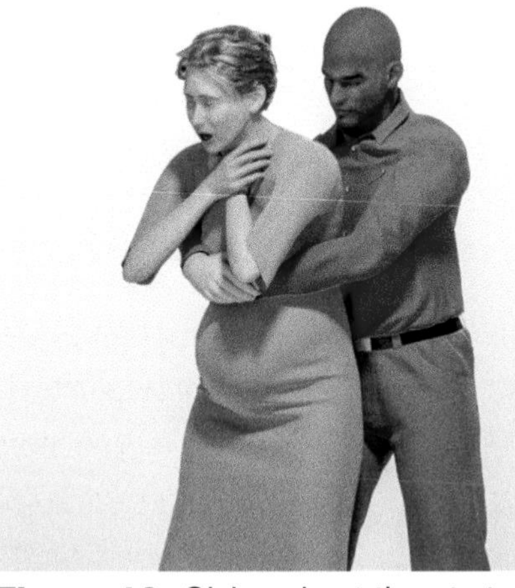

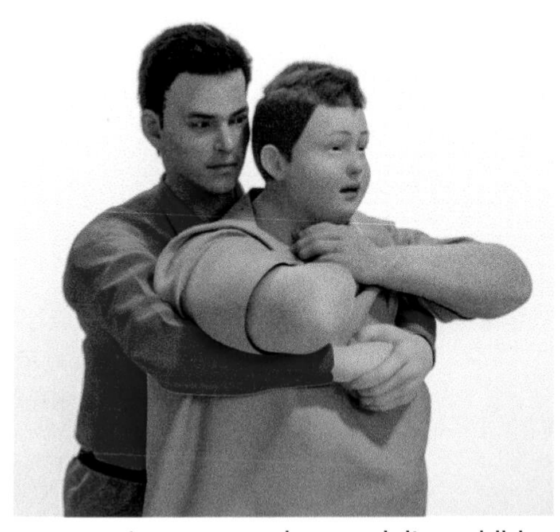

Figure 13. Giving chest thrusts to a choking pregnant woman or large adult or child.

How to Help a Choking Infant With a Severe Airway Block

When an infant has a severe airway block, use back slaps and chest thrusts to help remove the object. *Give only back slaps and chest thrusts to an infant who is choking.* Giving thrusts to an infant's abdomen can cause serious harm.

Follow these steps to help an infant who has a severe airway block:

How to Help a Choking Infant With a Severe Airway Block
☐ Hold the infant facedown on your forearm. Support the infant's head and jaw with your hand.
☐ Give up to 5 back slaps with the heel of your other hand, between the infant's shoulder blades (Figure 14A).
☐ If the object does not come out after 5 back slaps, turn the infant onto his back, supporting the head.
☐ Give up to 5 chest thrusts, using 2 fingers of your other hand to push on the chest in the same place you push during CPR (Figure 14B).
☐ Repeat giving 5 back slaps and 5 chest thrusts until the infant can breathe, cough, or cry, or until he becomes unresponsive.

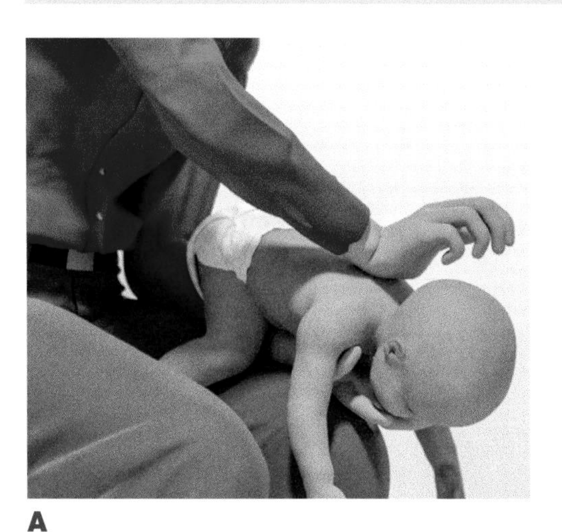

A

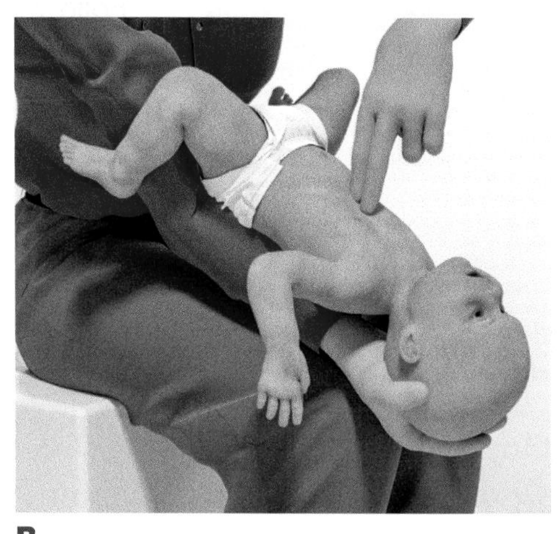

B

Figure 14. How to help an infant who has a severe airway block. **A,** Back slaps. **B,** Chest thrusts.

Help a Choking Adult, Child, or Infant Who Becomes Unresponsive

If you can't remove the object blocking the airway, the person will become unresponsive. Always give CPR to anyone who is unresponsive and not breathing normally or only gasping. Giving both compressions and breaths is very important for someone with a severe airway block who becomes unresponsive.

You will learn how to provide CPR and use an AED in the "CPR and AED" part of this workbook.

Remember	**Unresponsive + No breathing or only gasping = Provide CPR**

How to Help a Choking Adult Who Becomes Unresponsive

Follow these steps to help an adult with a severe airway block who becomes unresponsive:

How to Help a Choking Adult Who Becomes Unresponsive
☐ Shout for help.
☐ Phone or have someone else phone 9-1-1 and get an AED. Put the phone on speaker mode so that you can talk to the dispatcher.
☐ Provide CPR, starting with compressions.
☐ After each set of 30 compressions, open the airway to give breaths.
☐ Look in the mouth. If you see an object in the mouth, take it out.
☐ Give 2 breaths and then repeat 30 compressions.
☐ Continue CPR until • The person moves, speaks, blinks, or otherwise reacts • Someone with more advanced training arrives and takes over

Remember

Every time you open the airway to give breaths, look for the object in the back of the throat. If you see an object in the mouth, take it out.

Do not perform a blind finger sweep. This could cause the object to get lodged further back in the airway.

How to Help a Choking Child or Infant Who Becomes Unresponsive

A child or infant who has a severe airway block and becomes unresponsive needs immediate CPR. If you are alone without a cell phone, it is important to provide 5 sets of 30 compressions and 2 breaths first. Then, leave the child to phone 9-1-1 and get an AED if one is available.

Follow these steps to help a child or infant with a severe airway block who becomes unresponsive:

How to Help a Choking Child or Infant Who Becomes Unresponsive
☐ Shout for help. Make sure the child or infant is lying on his back on a firm, flat surface.
☐ Begin CPR, phone 9-1-1, and get an AED. *If someone comes to help and a cell phone is available* • Ask the person to phone 9-1-1 on the cell phone, put it on speaker mode, and go get an AED while you begin CPR.

(continued)

(continued)

How to Help a Choking Child or Infant Who Becomes Unresponsive

If someone comes to help and a cell phone is not available

- Ask the person to phone 9-1-1 and go get an AED while you begin CPR.

If you are alone and do have a cell phone or nearby phone

- Phone 9-1-1 and put the phone on speaker mode while you begin CPR.
- Give 5 sets of 30 compressions and 2 breaths.
- Go get an AED.*
- Return to the child or infant and continue CPR.

If you are alone and don't have a cell phone

- Give 5 sets of 30 compressions and 2 breaths.
- Phone 9-1-1 and get an AED.*
- Return to the child or infant and continue CPR.

*If the small child or infant isn't injured and you're alone, after 5 sets of 30 compressions and 2 breaths, you may carry him with you to phone 9-1-1 and get an AED.

☐ Provide CPR.

- Give sets of 30 compressions and 2 breaths.
- After each set of 30 compressions, open the airway to give breaths.
- Look in the mouth (Figure 15). If you see an object in the mouth, take it out.
- Give 2 breaths.

☐ Continue CPR and looking in the mouth after each set of compressions until

- The child or infant moves, cries, speaks, blinks, or otherwise reacts
- Someone with more advanced training arrives and takes over

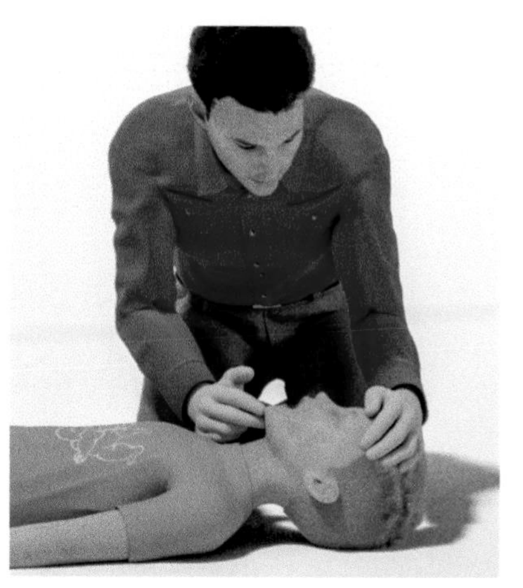

Figure 15. Look in the mouth for objects.

Allergic Reactions

Allergies are quite common. A severe allergic reaction can quickly turn into a medical emergency.

Some things that can cause a severe allergic reaction are

- Eggs
- Peanuts
- Chocolate
- Some medications
- Insect bites and stings, especially bee stings

Mild vs Severe Allergic Reaction

Allergic reactions can be mild or severe. However, some reactions that seem mild can become severe within minutes. Here are some signs of mild and severe allergic reactions:

Mild Allergic Reaction	Severe Allergic Reaction
• A stuffy nose, sneezing, and itching around the eyes	• Trouble breathing
• Itching of the skin	• Swelling of the tongue and face
• Raised, red rash on the skin (hives)	• Signs of shock

Epinephrine Pen for a Severe Allergic Reaction

Epinephrine is a drug that can stop a severe allergic reaction. It is available by prescription in a self-injectable pen device called an *epinephrine pen*. People who are known to have severe allergic reactions are encouraged to carry epinephrine pens with them at all times.

There are 2 types of epinephrine pens—spring activated and electronic. They are different for children and adults. So, be sure you are using the correct prescribed device.

If a person has an epinephrine pen, he will generally know how and when to use it. You may help give the person the injection if you have been trained and your state and employer allow it. The epinephrine injection is given in the side of the thigh.

How to Use an Epinephrine Pen

A severe allergic reaction can be life threatening. Follow these steps to help someone with signs of a severe allergic reaction use his epinephrine pen:

How to Use an Epinephrine Pen

- ☐ Follow the instructions on the pen. Make sure you are holding the pen in your fist without touching either end because the needle comes out of one end. You may give the injection through clothes or on bare skin.
- ☐ Take off the safety cap (Figure 16A).
- ☐ Hold the leg firmly in place just before and during the injection. Press the tip of the injector hard against the side of the person's thigh, about halfway between the hip and the knee (Figure 16B).
- ☐ For EpiPen and EpiPen Jr injectors, hold the injector in place for 3 seconds. Some other injectors may be held in place for up to 10 seconds. Be familiar with the manufacturer's instructions for the type of injector you are using.
- ☐ Pull the pen straight out, making sure you don't put your fingers over the end that has been pressed against the person's thigh.
- ☐ Either the person getting the injection or the person giving the injection should rub the injection spot for about 10 seconds.
- ☐ Note the time of the injection. Give the pen to the emergency responders for proper disposal.
- ☐ Call 9-1-1 if the person doesn't get better or if there is a delay greater than 10 minutes for advanced help to arrive. Consider giving a second dose, if available.

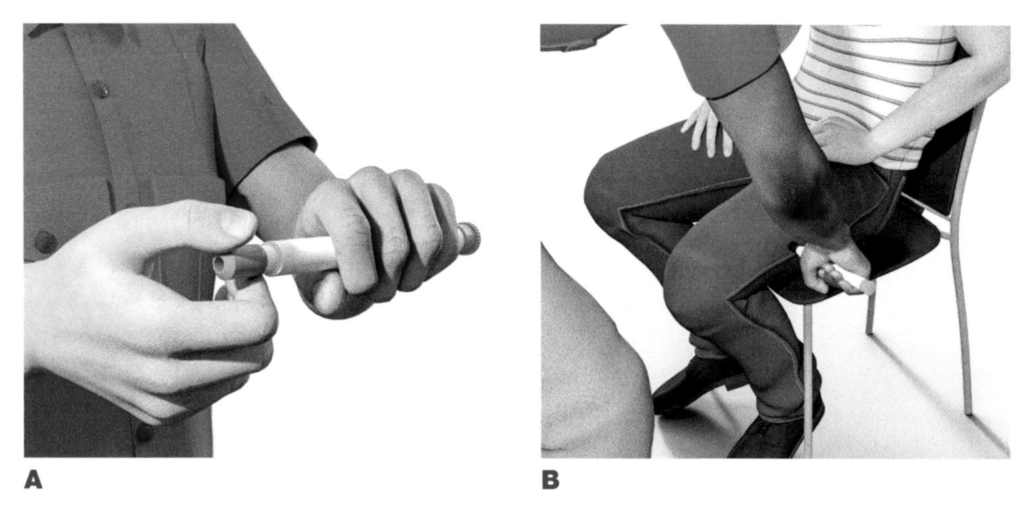

Figure 16. Using an epinephrine pen. **A,** Take off the safety cap. **B,** Press the tip of the injector hard against the side of the person's thigh, about halfway between the hip and the knee.

Dispose of the Epinephrine Pen Correctly

It's important to dispose of needles correctly so that no one gets stuck. Follow your company's sharps disposal policy. If you don't know what to do, give the needle to someone with more advanced training.

If possible, save a sample of what caused the reaction.

Heart Attack

Heart disease is the leading cause of death in the world.

If someone has signs of a possible heart attack, you must act and phone 9-1-1 right away—even if the person doesn't want you to. The first minutes of a heart attack are the most important. That's when a person is likely to get worse or even die. Also, many of the treatments for heart attack will be most successful if they are given quickly.

If a person says she has chest pain, make sure she stays calm and rests. It's best if the person doesn't drive herself to the hospital. Stay with her until someone with more advanced training arrives and takes over.

Life Is Why

Education Is Why

Heart disease is the No. 1 cause of death in the world—with more than 17 million deaths per year. That's why the AHA is continuously transforming our training solutions as science evolves, and driving awareness of how everyone can help save a life.

Difference Between Heart Attack and Cardiac Arrest

People often use the terms *sudden cardiac arrest* and *heart attack* to mean the same thing—but they are not the same.

- *Sudden cardiac arrest* is a "rhythm" problem. It occurs when the heart malfunctions and stops beating unexpectedly.
- A *heart attack* is a "clot" problem. It occurs when a clot blocks blood flow.

Sudden Cardiac Arrest

Sudden cardiac arrest results from an abnormal heart rhythm. This abnormal rhythm causes the heart to quiver so that it can no longer pump blood to the brain, lungs, and other organs.

Within seconds, the person becomes unresponsive and is not breathing or is only gasping. Death occurs within minutes if the victim does not receive immediate lifesaving treatment.

Heart Attack

A heart attack occurs when blood flow to part of the heart muscle is blocked by a clot. Typically, during a heart attack, the heart continues to pump blood.

A person having a heart attack may have discomfort or pain in the chest. There may be an uncomfortable feeling in one or both arms, the neck, the jaw, or the back between the shoulder blades.

The longer the person with a heart attack goes without treatment, the greater the possible damage to the heart muscle. Occasionally, the damaged heart muscle triggers an abnormal rhythm that can lead to sudden cardiac arrest.

Signs of a Heart Attack

Typical signs of a heart attack include the following:

Chest discomfort	Most heart attacks involve discomfort in the center of the chest that lasts more than a few minutes or that goes away and comes back. It can feel like uncomfortable pressure, squeezing, fullness, or pain.
Discomfort in other areas of the body	Discomfort also may appear in other areas of the upper body. Symptoms can include pain or discomfort in one or both arms, the back, neck, jaw, or stomach.
Other signs	Other signs of a heart attack are shortness of breath (with or without chest discomfort), breaking out in a cold sweat, nausea, or light-headedness.

Less Typical Signs in Women, the Elderly, and People With Diabetes

Women, the elderly, and people with diabetes are more likely to have less typical signs of a heart attack. These may include

- An ache in the chest, heartburn, or indigestion
- An uncomfortable feeling in the back, jaw, neck, or shoulder
- Shortness of breath
- Nausea or vomiting

Admitting Discomfort

Many people won't admit that their discomfort may be caused by a heart attack. People often say the following:

- "I'm too healthy."
- "I don't want to bother the doctor."
- "I don't want to frighten my spouse."
- "I'll feel silly if it isn't a heart attack."

If you suspect someone is having a heart attack, act quickly and phone 9-1-1 right away. Don't hesitate, even if the person doesn't want to admit discomfort.

Actions to Help Someone With Signs of a Heart Attack

Follow these first aid action steps if someone has any signs of a possible heart attack:

Actions to Help Someone With Signs of a Heart Attack
☐ Make sure the person stays calm and rests. Phone or have someone phone 9-1-1.
☐ Ask someone to get the first aid kit and AED if available.
☐ If the person has no allergy to aspirin, no serious bleeding, and no signs of a stroke, have the person chew and swallow 1 adult or 2 low-dose aspirins. • If the first aid provider is uncertain or uncomfortable with giving aspirin, the first aid provider should not encourage the person to take aspirin.
☐ If the person becomes unresponsive, be prepared to give CPR.

Fainting

Fainting is a short period of time, usually less than a minute, when a person briefly stops responding and then seems fine. Often, a person who faints gets dizzy and then becomes unresponsive.

Fainting may occur when someone

- Stands without moving for a long time, especially if it's hot
- Has a heart condition
- Suddenly stands after squatting or bending down
- Receives bad news

Actions to Help a Person Who May Faint

Follow these first aid action steps if a person is dizzy but still responds:

Actions to Help a Person Who May Faint
☐ Help the person lie flat on the floor.
☐ Phone 9-1-1 if the person doesn't improve or becomes unresponsive.
☐ If the person becomes unresponsive, give CPR.

Actions to Help a Person Who Has Fainted and Is Responsive

Follow these first aid action steps if a person faints and then starts to respond:

Actions to Help a Person Who Has Fainted and Is Responsive
☐ Ask the person to continue to lie flat on the floor until he can sit up and feels normal.
☐ If the person fell, look for injuries caused by the fall.
☐ Phone 9-1-1.

Diabetes and Low Blood Sugar

Diabetes is a disease that affects the levels of sugar in the blood. Too much or too little sugar causes problems. Some people with diabetes take medication, such as insulin, to maintain their sugar levels.

Low blood sugar can occur if a person with diabetes has not eaten or is vomiting, has not eaten enough food for the level of activity, or has injected too much insulin.

Signs of Low Blood Sugar in a Person With Diabetes

If the person's blood sugar does get too low, behavior can change. Signs of low blood sugar can come on quickly. When a person with diabetes has low blood sugar, the person may become

- Irritable or confused
- Hungry, thirsty, or weak
- Sleepy
- Sweaty

In some cases, the person might even have a seizure.

Actions to Take for a Responsive Person Who Has Low Blood Sugar

Follow these first aid action steps if the person is responsive and shows signs of low blood sugar:

Actions to Take for a Responsive Person Who Has Low Blood Sugar
If the person can't sit up or swallow
☐ Phone or have someone phone 9-1-1. Do not try to give the person anything to eat or drink.
If the person can sit up and swallow
☐ Ask the person to eat or drink something with sugar that can rapidly restore blood glucose levels. These items include glucose tablets, orange juice, soft chewy candy, jelly beans, fruit leather, or whole milk. ☐ Have the person sit quietly or lie down. ☐ If the person does not improve within 15 minutes, phone or have someone phone 9-1-1.

Stroke

Stroke is another medical emergency for which you may need to use your first aid skills. Strokes occur when blood stops flowing to a part of the brain. This can happen if a blood vessel in the brain is blocked or leaks.

Many people can be given treatments in the first hours after a stroke that can reduce the damage and improve recovery. Therefore, it's important to recognize the signs of stroke quickly and get immediate medical care.

Warning Signs of Stroke

You can use the FAST method to recognize and remember the warning signs of stroke. *FAST* stands for face, arms, speech, and time.

F	***F**ace drooping:* Does one side of the face droop or is it numb?
A	***A**rm weakness:* Is one arm weak or numb?
S	***S**peech difficulty:* Is speech slurred?
T	***T**ime to phone 9-1-1:* If someone shows any of these symptoms, phone 9-1-1 immediately.

Actions to Help a Person Who May Have Had a Stroke

Follow these first aid action steps if you think someone is having a stroke:

Actions to Help a Person Who May Have Had a Stroke
☐ Phone or have someone phone 9-1-1 and get the first aid kit and AED.
☐ Note the time when the stroke signs first appeared.
☐ Remain with the person until someone with more advanced training arrives and takes over.
☐ If the person becomes unresponsive and is not breathing normally or only gasping, give CPR.

Seizure

A seizure is abnormal electrical activity in the brain. Most seizures stop within a few minutes and are often caused by a medical condition called epilepsy. Seizures also can be caused by head injury, low blood sugar, heat-related injury, poisoning, or sudden cardiac arrest.

Signs of a Seizure

Signs of a seizure may differ. Some people who are having a seizure may

- Lose muscle control
- Have jerking movement of the arms, legs, and sometimes other parts of the body
- Fall to the ground
- Stop responding

However, not all seizures look like this. Other people might become unresponsive and have a glassy-eyed stare.

During the seizure, a person may bite her tongue, cheek, or mouth. You can give first aid for that injury after the seizure is over. After a seizure, it isn't unusual for the person to be slow to respond or confused, or even to fall asleep.

Caution

The most important first aid action for a person having a seizure is to protect the person from injury.

There are some myths about what you should do to help someone who is having a seizure. Some of these can actually harm a person instead of helping. The correct information for how to help a person who is having a seizure is discussed in this workbook and during the course.

Actions to Help a Person Who Is Having a Seizure

Follow these first aid action steps to help someone during a seizure:

Actions to Help a Person Who Is Having a Seizure
☐ Move furniture or other objects out of the way.
☐ Place a small pad or towel under the person's head.
☐ Phone 9-1-1 and get the first aid kit.

Actions to Help a Person After a Seizure

Follow these first aid action steps to help someone after a seizure:

Actions to Help a Person After a Seizure
☐ Quickly check to see if the person is responsive and breathing.
☐ Stay with the person until someone with more advanced training arrives and takes over. • If the person is having trouble breathing because of vomiting or fluids in her mouth, roll the person onto her side. • If she is unresponsive and is not breathing normally or only gasping, give CPR.

Bleeding From the Mouth

If the person has bitten her tongue, cheek, or mouth and is bleeding, give first aid after the seizure. See “Bleeding From the Mouth” in “Part 4: Injury Emergencies.”

Medical Emergencies: Review Questions

Question	Your Notes
1. When giving abdominal thrusts to an adult who is choking, you should a. Place your hands near the throat b. Place your hands near the left side of the lower abdomen c. Put the thumb side of your fist slightly above her navel (belly button) and well below the breastbone	
2. Signs of a severe allergic reaction include trouble breathing, swelling of the face and tongue, and the person may stop responding. True False	
3. A person with a _____________ is usually awake and can talk but may have an uncomfortable feeling, such as pain or pressure, in the chest. a. Stroke b. Seizure c. Heart attack	
4. The warning signs of __________ include sudden numbness or weakness of the face, arm, or leg, especially on one side of the body. a. Fainting b. Stroke c. Heart attack d. Seizure	
5. If someone with low blood sugar is responding and can sit up and swallow, give her something that contains sugar to eat or drink. True False	

Answers: **1.** c, **2.** True, **3.** c, **4.** b, **5.** True

Part 3: Injury Emergencies

The injuries discussed in this section are those you are most likely to encounter. In some cases, the injury may not seem urgent, but some injuries can become serious if not treated.

Topics Covered

Topics covered in this part are

- External bleeding
- Wounds
- Internal bleeding
- Head, neck, and spinal injuries
- Broken bones and sprains
- Burns and electrical injuries

As you read and study this part, pay particular attention to the skills that you may be asked to demonstrate during the course:

- Controlling bleeding by direct pressure and bandaging
- Splinting (optional)

External Bleeding

Bleeding can be either external or internal. Bleeding can quickly become life threatening if not controlled.

Severe bleeding occurs when a large blood vessel is cut or torn. When this happens, a person can lose a lot of blood within minutes.

Minor bleeding occurs from small cuts or scrapes. Most bleeding can be stopped with pressure. It's important to stay calm. Bleeding often looks worse than it is.

Dressing vs Bandage

Many people confuse the terms *dressing* and *bandage*. Here is what they mean and how they work together:

- A *dressing* is a clean material used directly on a wound to stop bleeding. It can be a piece of gauze or any other clean piece of cloth.
- A *bandage* is material used to protect or cover an injured body part. A bandage may also be used to help keep pressure on a wound.

If necessary, you can hold gauze dressings in place over a wound with a bandage (Figure 17).

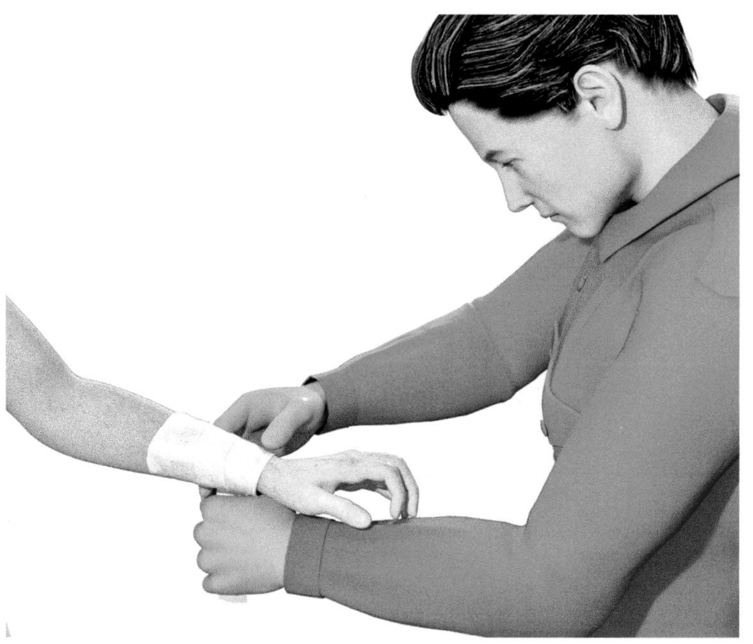

Figure 17. Placing a bandage over a dressing.

When to Phone 9-1-1 for Bleeding

Phone or ask someone to phone 9-1-1 if

- There is a lot of bleeding
- You cannot stop the bleeding
- You see signs of shock
- You suspect a head, neck, or spine injury
- You are not sure what to do

Control Bleeding by Direct Pressure and Bandaging

Actions to Control Bleeding

Follow these first aid action steps to help someone who is bleeding:

Actions to Control Bleeding
☐ Make sure the scene is safe.
☐ Send someone to get the first aid kit.
☐ Put on PPE.
☐ If possible, have the person apply direct pressure to the wound while you put on your PPE.

(continued)

(continued)

Actions to Control Bleeding
☐ Apply dressings from the first aid kit. Put direct pressure on the dressings over the bleeding area. Use the flat part of your fingers or the palm of your hand (Figure 18).
☐ If the bleeding doesn't stop, you'll need to add a second dressing and press harder. Do not remove a dressing once it's in place because this could cause the wound to bleed more. Keep pressure on the wound until it stops bleeding.
☐ Once the bleeding has stopped or if you can't keep pressure on the wound, wrap a bandage firmly over the dressings to hold them in place.
☐ For minor cuts, wash the area with soap and water. Then, apply a dressing to the wound.

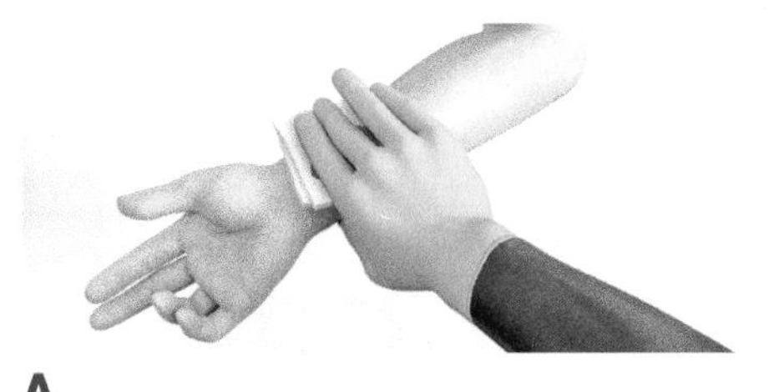

A

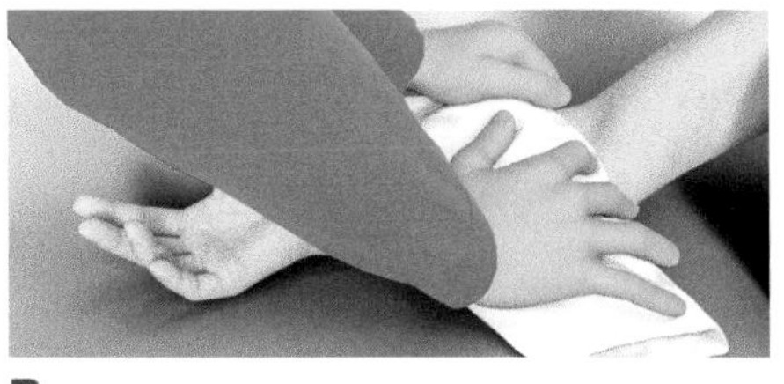

B

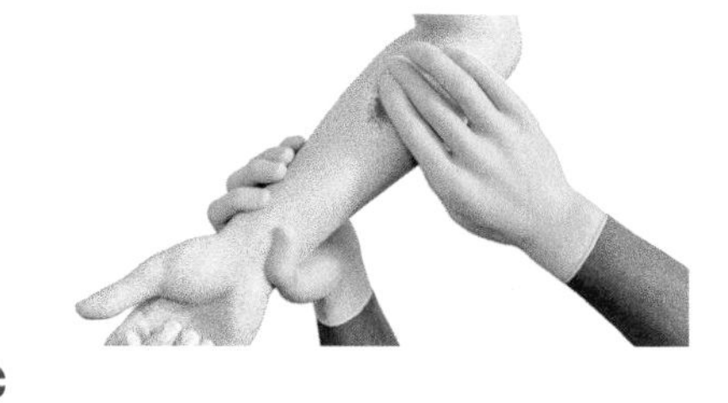

C

Figure 18. Controlling bleeding. **A,** A dressing can be a gauze pad or pads. **B,** It can be any other clean piece of cloth. **C,** If you do not have a dressing, use your gloved hand.

Use a Tourniquet

If an arm or leg has severe bleeding and you can't stop the bleeding with direct pressure, you can use a tourniquet. You should make sure you call 9-1-1 and get an AED, if available, because uncontrolled bleeding can lead to more complications.

The first aid kit should contain a premade or manufactured tourniquet. It includes a strap that you wrap around the injured person's arm or leg and a straight, stick-like object called a windlass. The windlass is used to tighten the tourniquet. If applied correctly, a tourniquet should stop the bleeding.

If you apply the tourniquet correctly, it will cause pain as it stops the bleeding.

Once you have the tourniquet in place, note the time and leave it alone until someone with more advanced training arrives and takes over.

Actions to Apply a Premade Tourniquet

Follow these first aid action steps to apply a premade tourniquet from your first aid kit (Figure 19):

Actions to Apply a Premade Tourniquet
☐ Make sure the scene is safe.
☐ Phone 9-1-1 and get the first aid kit (if you do not already have it) and an AED.
☐ Wear PPE.
☐ Place the tourniquet about 2 inches above the injury if possible.
☐ Tighten the tourniquet until the bleeding stops.
☐ Note what time the tourniquet was placed on the body.
☐ Once you have the tourniquet in place and the bleeding has stopped, leave it alone until someone with more advanced training arrives and takes over.

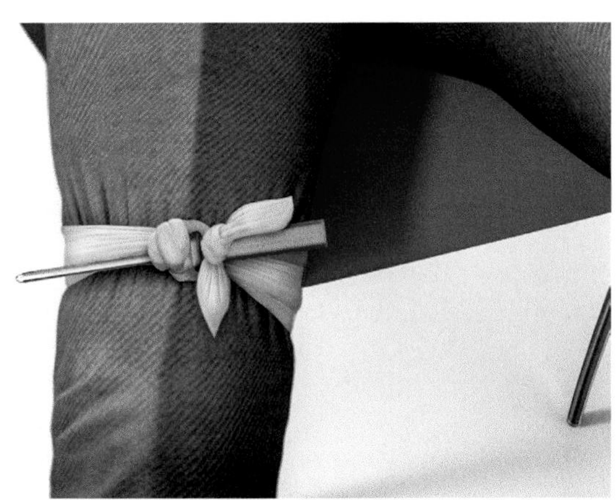

Figure 19. A tourniquet applied to a leg.

Actions to Make and Apply a Tourniquet

If you don't have a tourniquet, you can make one. Follow these actions to make and apply a tourniquet:

Actions to Make and Apply a Tourniquet
☐ Make sure the scene is safe.
☐ Phone 9-1-1 and get the first aid kit (if you do not already have it) and an AED.
☐ Wear PPE.
☐ Fold a cloth or bandage so that it's long and at least 1 inch wide.

(continued)

(continued)

Actions to Make and Apply a Tourniquet
☐ Wrap the bandage 2 inches above the injury if possible.
☐ Tie the ends of the bandage around a small hand tool, stick, or something similar.
☐ Turn the item to tighten the tourniquet.
☐ Continue tightening until the bleeding stops.
☐ Secure the hand tool or stick so that the tourniquet stays tight.
☐ Note what time the tourniquet was placed.
☐ Once you have the tourniquet in place and the bleeding has stopped, leave it alone until someone with more advanced training arrives and takes over.

Shock

Losing a large amount of blood can lead to shock. Besides loss of blood, shock can be caused by other types of emergencies, such as a heart attack or severe allergic reaction.

Signs of Shock

A person in shock may

- Feel weak, faint, or dizzy
- Feel nauseated or thirsty
- Have pale or grayish skin
- Be restless, agitated, or confused
- Be cold and clammy to the touch

Actions to Help a Person in Shock

Follow these first aid action steps to help a person in shock (Figure 20):

Actions to Help a Person in Shock
☐ Make sure the scene is safe.
☐ Phone 9-1-1 and get the first aid kit and AED if available.
☐ Help the person lie on his back.
☐ Cover the person with a blanket to keep him warm.
☐ Check to see if CPR is needed. If so, give CPR.

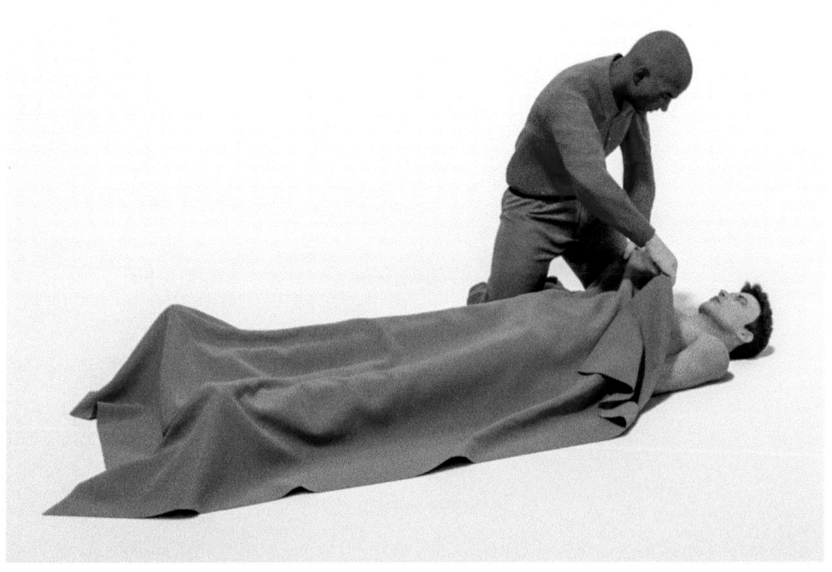

Figure 20. A person in shock.

Wounds

Wounds are common first aid emergencies. A wound is an injury of the soft tissue in the body. Wounds can range from minor, such as scrapes and small cuts, to more serious injuries.

Bleeding From the Nose

Actions to Help Someone With a Nosebleed

To stop a nosebleed, apply pressure. Follow these first aid action steps:

Actions to Help Someone With a Nosebleed
☐ Make sure the scene is safe.
☐ Wear PPE.
☐ Have the person sit and lean forward.
☐ Pinch the soft part of the nose on both sides (Figure 21) with a clean dressing.
☐ Place constant pressure on the nostrils for a few minutes until the bleeding stops. If bleeding continues, press harder.
☐ Phone 9-1-1 if • You can't stop the bleeding in about 15 minutes • The bleeding is heavy, such as gushing blood • The injured person has trouble breathing

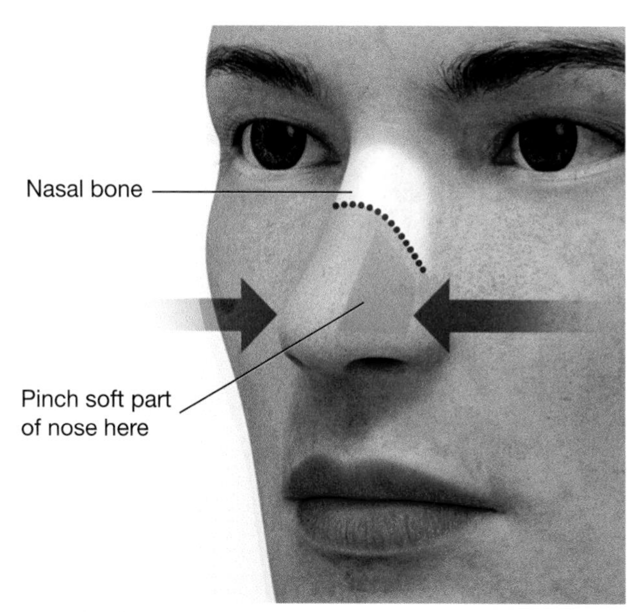

Figure 21. Press on both sides of the nostrils.

Leaning Forward

A person with a nosebleed should lean forward (not backward). Leaning backward will not help stop the bleeding. You will see less blood when a person tilts his head back, because the blood drains down the person's throat. Swallowed blood can lead to vomiting.

Bleeding From the Mouth

When a person has a mouth injury, it can be serious if blood or broken teeth block the airway and cause breathing problems.

Bleeding from the mouth can usually be stopped with pressure.

Actions to Help Someone With Bleeding From the Mouth

Follow these first aid action steps when giving first aid to a person with bleeding from the mouth:

Actions to Help Someone With Bleeding From the Mouth
☐ Make sure the scene is safe.
☐ Get the first aid kit.
☐ Wear PPE.
☐ If bleeding is coming from the tongue, lip, or cheek and you can reach it easily, apply pressure with gauze or a clean cloth (Figure 22).
☐ If you haven't phoned 9-1-1 and you can't stop the bleeding or the person has trouble breathing, phone or ask someone else to phone 9-1-1.

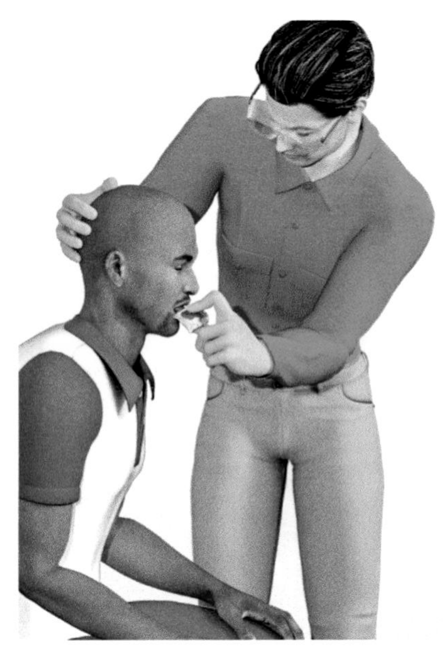

Figure 22. If the bleeding is from the tongue, lip, or cheek, press the bleeding area with sterile gauze or a clean cloth.

Tooth Injuries

Sometimes, when a person suffers a mouth injury, one or more teeth may be broken, become loose, or have been knocked out. This can be a choking hazard.

Actions to Help Someone With a Tooth Injury

Follow these steps when giving first aid to a person with a tooth injury:

Actions to Help Someone With a Tooth Injury
☐ Make sure the scene is safe.
☐ Get the first aid kit.
☐ Wear PPE.
☐ Check the person's mouth for any missing or loose teeth or parts of teeth.
☐ If a tooth is chipped, gently clean the injured area and call a dentist.
☐ If a tooth is loose, have the person bite down on a piece of gauze to keep the tooth in place, and call a dentist.
☐ If a tooth has come out, it may be possible for a dentist to reattach the tooth. So, when you hold it, hold it by the crown—the top part of the tooth (Figure 23). Do not hold it by the root.
☐ Apply pressure with gauze to stop any bleeding in the empty tooth socket.

(continued)

(continued)

Actions to Help Someone With a Tooth Injury
☐ Clean the area where the tooth was located with saline or clean water.
☐ Put the tooth in one of the following: egg white, coconut water, or whole milk.
☐ If none of these is available, store the tooth in the injured person's saliva—not in the mouth.
☐ Immediately take the injured person and tooth to a dentist or emergency department.

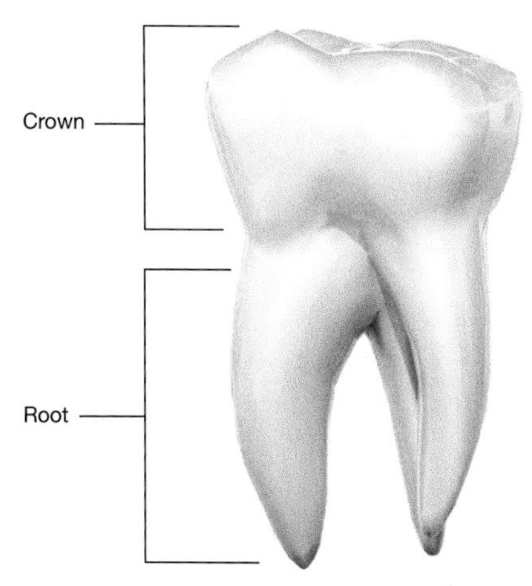

Figure 23. Hold the tooth by the crown.

Eye Injuries

Eye injuries are a fairly common first aid emergency. Any direct hit, such as a punch to the eye or chemical in the eye, can create big problems. If the eye is hit hard or punctured, phone 9-1-1 and tell the person to keep both eyes closed.

Signs of an Eye Injury

Signs of an eye injury include

- Pain
- Trouble seeing
- Bruising
- Bleeding
- Redness or swelling

Actions to Help Someone With an Eye Injury

Follow these first aid action steps to help someone with an eye injury:

Actions to Help Someone With an Eye Injury
☐ Make sure the scene is safe.
☐ Get the first aid kit.
☐ Wear PPE.
☐ If something small like sand gets in a person's eye, rinse with lots of running water.
☐ Phone 9-1-1 if • The sand or object doesn't come out • The person has extreme pain • The person still has trouble seeing
☐ Tell the person to keep his eyes closed until someone with more advanced training arrives and takes over.

Actions to Help Someone With a Toxic Eye Injury

Follow these first aid action steps if someone gets a toxic chemical in the eye:

Actions to Help Someone With a Toxic Eye Injury
☐ Make sure the scene is safe.
☐ Get the first aid kit.
☐ Wear PPE.
☐ If chemicals get in a person's eyes, rinse with lots of water (Figure 24). Rinse for at least 15 minutes or until someone with more advanced training arrives and takes over. • *Caution:* If only one eye is affected, make sure the eye with the chemicals in it is the lower eye as you rinse. Try not to rinse the chemicals into the unaffected eye.
☐ If an eyewash station is nearby or you have access to an eyewash kit, use it.
☐ If neither is available, use water from the tap or normal saline or contact lens solution.
☐ Phone 9-1-1.

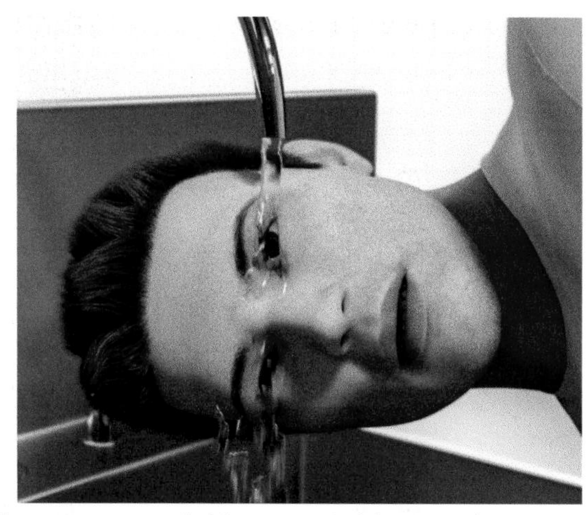

Figure 24. Help the person wash his eyes and face under water flowing from a faucet or hose, or use an eyewash station.

Penetrating and Puncturing Injuries

Penetrating and puncturing injuries to the body are treated differently from more common bleeding injuries.

An object such as a knife, nail, or sharp stick can wound a person by penetrating the body or puncturing the skin. If the object is stuck in the body, leave it there until a healthcare provider can treat the injury. Taking it out may cause more bleeding and damage.

Actions to Take for a Penetrating or Puncturing Injury

Follow these first aid action steps for penetrating and puncturing injuries:

Actions to Take for a Penetrating or Puncturing Injury
☐ Make sure the scene is safe.
☐ Phone or send someone to phone 9-1-1 and get the first aid kit and the AED.
☐ Wear PPE.
☐ Try to stop any bleeding you can see. Do not try to remove the object if it is stuck in the body.

Amputation

One external bleeding injury that may seem overwhelming is traumatic amputation.

Amputation occurs when any part of an arm or leg is cut or torn off. It may be possible to reattach amputated fingers or toes. Because of this, it's important to know first aid actions to first stop bleeding by using pressure and possibly a tourniquet and then to protect the amputated part.

Actions to Give First Aid to a Person With an Amputation

Follow these first aid action steps when giving first aid to a person with an amputation:

Actions to Give First Aid to a Person With an Amputation
☐ Make sure the scene is safe.
☐ Phone or send someone to phone 9-1-1 and get the first aid kit and the AED.
☐ Wear PPE.
☐ Stop the bleeding from the injured area with pressure. You may have to press for a long time with very firm pressure to stop the bleeding.
☐ If you find the amputated part, follow the "Actions to Protect an Amputated Part" section.

Actions to Protect an Amputated Part

Follow these first aid action steps to protect an amputated part:

Actions to Protect an Amputated Part
☐ Make sure the scene is safe.
☐ Rinse the amputated part with clean water (Figure 25A).
☐ Cover it with a clean dressing.
☐ Place it in a watertight plastic bag (Figure 25B).
☐ Place the bag in another container with ice or ice and water (Figure 25C). Label it with the injured person's name, the date, and the time.
☐ Make sure the body part gets to the hospital with the injured person. *Remember:* Do not place the amputated body part directly on ice because extreme cold can injure it.

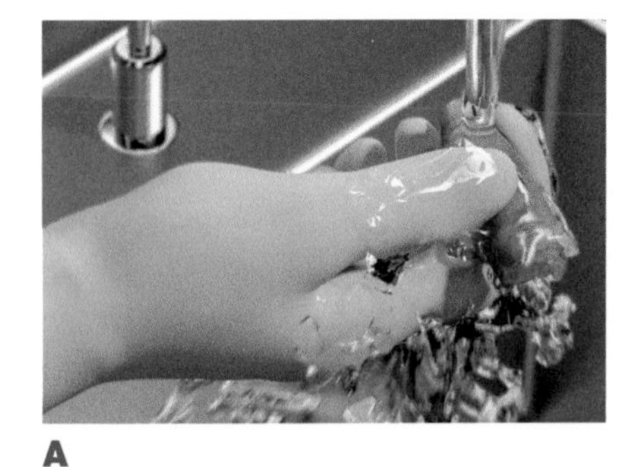

A

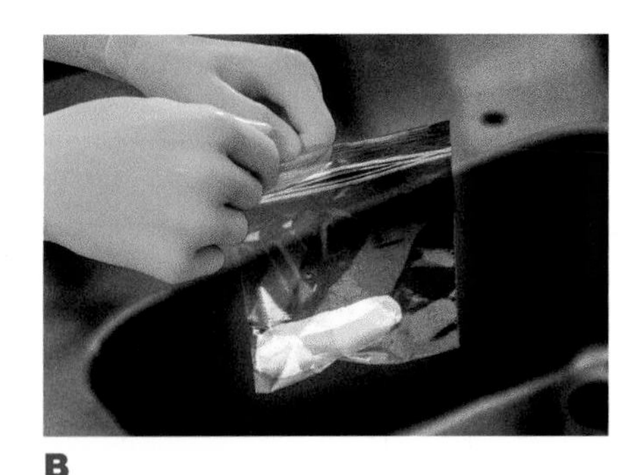

B

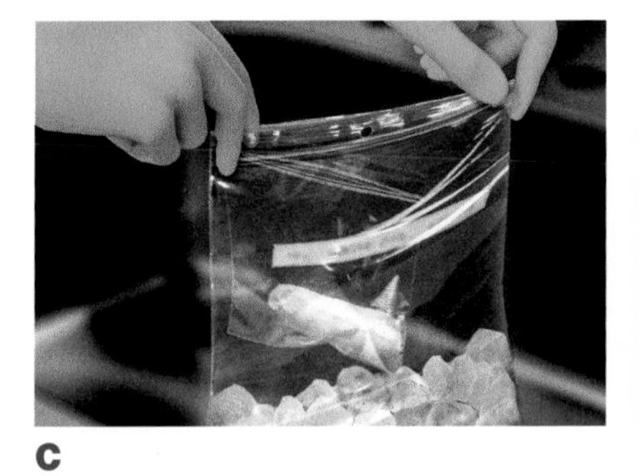

C

Figure 25. A, If you can find the amputated part, rinse it with clean water. **B,** If it will fit, place the wrapped part in a watertight plastic bag. **C,** Place that bag in another labeled bag with ice or ice water.

Internal Bleeding

Internal bleeding is bleeding inside the body. When bleeding occurs inside the body, you may be able to see a bruise under the skin, or you may not see any signs at all. When bleeding is internal, you can't tell how much bleeding has occurred.

Signs of Internal Bleeding

You should suspect internal bleeding if a person has

- An injury from a car crash, been hit by a car, or fallen from a height
- An injury in the abdomen or chest (including bruises such as seat belt marks)
- Sports injuries, such as slamming into other people or being hit with a ball
- Pain in the abdomen or chest after an injury
- Shortness of breath after an injury
- Coughed up or vomited blood after an injury
- Signs of shock without external bleeding
- A knife or a gunshot wound

Actions to Help a Person With Suspected Internal Bleeding

If you suspect internal bleeding, follow these first aid action steps:

Actions to Help a Person With Suspected Internal Bleeding
☐ Make sure the scene is safe.
☐ Phone or send someone to phone 9-1-1 and get the first aid kit and the AED.
☐ Wear PPE.
☐ Have the person lie down and keep still.
☐ Check for signs of shock.
☐ Give CPR if needed.

Head, Neck, and Spinal Injuries

With any kind of head, neck, or spinal injury, be cautious about moving an injured person.

Suspect a head, neck, or spinal injury if the person

- Fell from a height
- Was injured by a strong blow to the head
- Was injured while diving
- Was involved in a car crash
- Was riding a bicycle or motorbike involved in a crash, especially when not wearing a helmet or the helmet broke in the crash

Signs of a Head Injury

Suspect a head injury if an injured person

- Does not respond or only moans
- Acts sleepy or confused
- Vomits
- Has trouble seeing, walking, or moving any part of the body
- Has a seizure

If a person has a head injury that results in a change in consciousness, worsening signs or symptoms, or other cause for concern, the person should be evaluated by a healthcare provider or EMS personnel as soon as possible. Phone 9-1-1 if the person becomes unresponsive.

A person with these signs should not play sports, drive a car, ride a bike, or work with heavy machinery until a healthcare provider says it's OK to do so.

Concussion

A concussion is a type of head injury. Concussions usually happen because of falls, motor vehicle accidents, and sports injuries. A concussion may occur when the head or body is hit so hard that the brain moves inside the skull.

Possible signs of concussion are

- Feeling stunned or dazed
- Confusion
- Headache
- Nausea or vomiting
- Dizziness, unsteadiness, or difficulty in balance
- Double vision or flashing lights
- Loss of memory of events that happened before or after the injury

Spinal Injury

If a person falls, an injury to the spine is possible. The spine protects the spinal cord.

Suspect possible spinal damage if an injured person

- Was in a car or bicycle crash
- Has fallen
- Has tingling or is weak in the extremities
- Has pain or tenderness in the neck or back
- Appears intoxicated or not fully alert
- Is 65 years of age or older
- Has other painful injuries, especially to the head or neck

Caution

When a person has a spinal injury, *do not twist or turn the head or neck* unless it's necessary to do any of the following:

- Turn the person faceup to give CPR
- Move the person out of danger
- Reposition the person because of breathing problems, vomiting, or fluids in the mouth

---

Actions to Help a Person With a Possible Head, Neck, or Spinal Injury

Follow these first aid action steps when giving first aid to a person with a possible head, neck, or spinal injury:

Actions to Help a Person With a Possible Head, Neck, or Spinal Injury
☐ Make sure the scene is safe.
☐ Phone or send someone to phone 9-1-1 and get the first aid kit and the AED.
☐ Have the person remain as still as possible. Wait for someone with more advanced training to arrive and take over.
☐ Do not twist or turn the person's head or neck unless absolutely necessary.

With this type of injury, you may have to control external bleeding. This is why it is important to get the first aid kit. Getting the AED is also important in case the person's condition worsens and you need to give CPR before someone with more advanced training arrives and takes over.

Broken Bones and Sprains

Injuries to bones, joints, and muscles are common. But without an x-ray, it may be impossible to tell whether a bone is broken or the injury is a sprain. Either way, you'll take the same first aid actions.

Actions to Take for a Person With a Possible Broken Bone or Sprain

Follow these first aid action steps for a person with a possible broken bone or sprain:

Actions to Take for a Person With a Possible Broken Bone or Sprain
☐ Make sure the scene is safe.
☐ Get the first aid kit.
☐ Wear PPE.
☐ Cover any open wound with a clean dressing.
☐ Put a towel on top of the injured body part. Place a bag filled with ice and water on top of the towel over the injured area (Figure 26). Keep the ice in place for up to 20 minutes.
☐ Phone 9-1-1 if • There is a large open wound • The injured body part is abnormally bent • You're not sure what to do
☐ If the injured body part hurts, the person should avoid using it until checked by a healthcare provider.

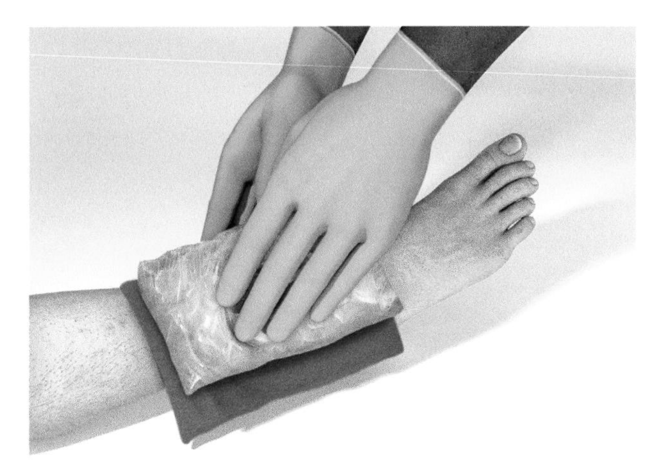

Figure 26. Put a plastic bag filled with ice and water on the injured area with a towel between the bag and the skin.

A splint keeps an injured body part from moving. If a broken bone has come through the skin or is bent, it shouldn't be straightened. The injury needs to be protected until someone with more advanced training arrives and takes over.

Caution

If the injured part is bleeding, apply direct pressure to stop the bleeding. Apply a dressing to the wound before applying the splint.

Leave bent and deformed body parts in their bent or deformed positions as you apply the splint. If a broken bone has come through the skin, cover the wound with a clean dressing and splint as needed.

Actions to Apply a Splint

Follow these first aid action steps to apply a splint:

Actions to Apply a Splint
☐ Make sure the scene is safe.
☐ Get the first aid kit.
☐ Wear PPE.
☐ Find an object that you can use to keep the injured arm or leg from moving.
☐ Rolled-up towels, magazines, and pieces of wood can be used as splints. Splint in a way to reduce pain and limit further injury. The splint should be longer than the injured area and should support the joints above and below the injury (Figure 27).
☐ After covering any broken skin with a clean or sterile cloth, tie or tape the splint to the injured limb so that it supports the injured area.
☐ Use tape, gauze, or cloth to secure it. It should fit snugly but not cut off circulation.
☐ If you're using a hard splint, like wood, make sure you pad it with something soft, like clothing or a towel.
☐ Keep the limb still until the injured person can be seen by a healthcare provider.

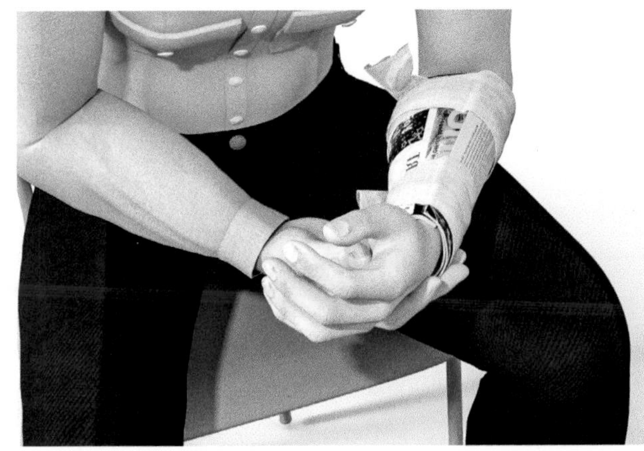

Figure 27. Use stiff material, such as a rolled-up magazine, to splint injured body parts.

Actions to Take to Self-Splint an Arm

If you don't have anything to use as a splint, a person can use his other arm to hold the injured one in place. Follow these steps to self-splint an arm:

Actions to Take to Self-Splint an Arm
☐ Have the injured person place his hand across his chest and hold it in place with his other arm.

Burns and Electrical Injuries

Burns

Burns are injuries that can be caused by contact with heat, electricity, or chemicals. Specifically, heat burns are caused when a person comes in contact with a hot surface, hot liquids, steam, or fire.

The only thing you should put on a burn is cool water and clean dressings—never use ice. It can actually damage a burned area. Follow any further instructions by a healthcare provider.

Actions to Take for Small Burns

Follow these first aid action steps for small burns:

Actions to Take for Small Burns
☐ Make sure the scene is safe.
☐ Get the first aid kit.
☐ Wear PPE.
☐ Cool the burn area immediately with cold, but not ice-cold, water for at least 10 minutes (Figure 28).

(continued)

(continued)

Actions to Take for Small Burns
☐ If you do not have cold water, use a cool or cold, but not freezing, clean compress.
☐ Run cold water on the burn until it doesn't hurt.
☐ You may cover the burn with a dry, nonstick sterile or clean dressing.

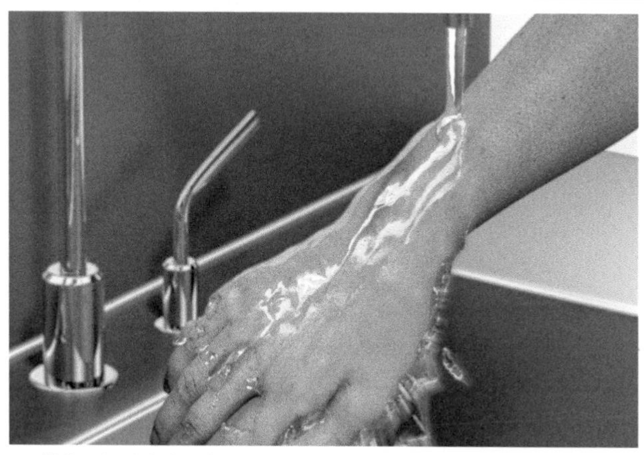

Figure 28. If possible, hold the burned area under cold running water.

Actions to Take for Large Burns

Follow these first aid action steps for large burns:

Actions to Take for Large Burns
☐ Make sure the scene is safe.
☐ If there is a fire, the burn area is large, or you're not sure what to do, phone 9-1-1.
☐ If the person or his clothing is on fire, put the fire out. Have the person stop, drop, and roll. Then, cover the person with a wet blanket.
☐ Once the fire is out, remove the wet blanket. Carefully remove jewelry and clothing that is not stuck to the skin.
☐ For large burns, cool the burn area immediately with cold water for at least 10 minutes.
☐ After you cool the burns, cover them with dry, nonstick, sterile or clean dressings.
☐ Cover the person with a dry blanket.

(continued)

(continued)

Actions to Take for Large Burns
☐ Check for signs of shock.
☐ A person with a large burn should be seen by a healthcare provider as soon as possible.
☐ A healthcare provider can determine if additional treatment is necessary.

Electrical Injuries

Electricity can cause burns on the outside of the body and on the inside, injuring organs. You may see marks or wounds where the electricity has entered and left the body. The damage can be severe, but there's no way to tell how severe based on the marks on the outside. Electricity can stop breathing or cause a deadly abnormal heart rhythm and cardiac arrest.

If an electrical injury is caused by high voltage, like a fallen power line, immediately notify the proper authorities, and phone 9-1-1. Don't enter the area or try to move wires until the power has been turned off.

Caution

Electricity can travel from the power source through the person to you. Because of this, don't touch a person if he is still in contact with the power source. It's best to turn the power off, but only attempt this if you are trained to do so. Once the power is off, you may touch the injured person.

Actions to Take for an Electrical Injury

Follow these first aid action steps for someone with an electrical injury:

Actions to Take for an Electrical Injury
☐ Make sure the scene is safe.
☐ Get the first aid kit and AED.
☐ Wear PPE.
☐ Phone 9-1-1.
☐ When it is safe to touch the injured person, give CPR if it is needed.
☐ A healthcare provider should check anyone who has an electrical injury as soon as possible.

Injury Emergencies: Review Questions

Question	Your Notes
1. To help stop bleeding that you can see, put firm pressure on a dressing or bandage over the bleeding area. True False	
2. *Mark an X by the correct response.* A person with a nosebleed should lean ____ forward. ____ backward.	
3. *Mark an X by the correct response.* If a large stick or a knife has been pushed into someone's body, you should ____ remove it as quickly as possible. ____ leave it in and get help.	
4. If someone falls down and then becomes sleepy or confused, vomits, or complains of a headache, the person may have a head injury. True False	
5. As soon as a person twists his ankle, apply a heating pad or heat pack over the injured area for 20 minutes to help reduce swelling. True False	
6. To give first aid for a small burn on the arm, cool the burn with a. lukewarm water. b. ice directly on the skin. c. cold, but not ice-cold, water.	

Answers: **1.** True, **2.** Forward, **3.** Leave it in, **4.** True, **5.** False, **6.** c

Part 4: Environmental Emergencies

What You Will Learn

Topics covered in this part are

- Bites and stings
- Heat-related emergencies
- Cold-related emergencies
- Poison emergencies

Bites and Sting

Animal and Human Bites

When an animal bite breaks the skin, the wound can bleed and become infected.

Not only is the bite a concern, the risk of rabies from dogs or wild animals must be considered. Rabies in wild animals is most frequently reported in raccoons, skunks, and bats. Dogs bitten by infected animals can become infected.

Also, because of the risk of rabies, anyone who has had direct contact with a bat or has been alone in a room with a bat should contact a healthcare provider as soon as possible.

Actions to Take for an Animal or Human Bite

Follow these first aid action steps for a person with an animal or human bite:

Actions to Take for an Animal or Human Bite
☐ Make sure the scene is safe for you and the person who has been bitten.
☐ Get the first aid kit.
☐ Wear PPE.
☐ With animal bites, be sure to wash the wound with plenty of soap and water.
☐ Apply a bag of ice and water wrapped in a towel to help with bruising and swelling.
☐ If there is a bruise or swelling, place a bag of ice and water wrapped in a towel on the bite for up to 20 minutes.
☐ For all bites that break the skin, phone a healthcare provider as soon as possible.

Snakebites

If someone has been bitten by a snake, you can sometimes identify the snake from its color or bite mark. But if you're not sure, assume that the snake is poisonous.

Signs of poisonous snakebites are

- Pain at the bite area that keeps getting worse
- Swelling of the bite area
- Nausea, vomiting, sweating, or weakness

Scene Safety and Snakebites

When making sure the scene is safe, be very careful around any snake, even if it's wounded. Back away and go around the snake.

If the snake has been killed or hurt, don't handle it. A snake can bite even when severely hurt or close to death.

Actions to Take for a Snakebite

Follow these first aid action steps to help a person bitten by a snake:

Actions to Take for a Snakebite
☐ Make sure the scene is safe for you and the person who has been bitten.
☐ Get the first aid kit.
☐ Wear PPE.
☐ Ask another adult to move any other people away from the area and phone 9-1-1.
☐ Ask the injured person to stay as still and calm as possible and avoid moving the part of the body that was bitten.
☐ Remove any tight clothing and jewelry.
☐ Gently wash the area with running water and soap.
☐ Keep the person still and calm until someone with more advanced training arrives and takes over.

Insect, Bee, and Spider Bites and Stings

Usually, insect bites and stings cause only mild pain, itching, and swelling at the bite. However, some insect bites can be serious and even fatal if

- The person bitten has a severe allergic reaction to the bite or sting
- Poison (venom) is injected into the person from the bite or sting

Bees are the only insects that leave behind their stingers. If you or someone you know gets stung by a bee, you should look for the stinger and remove it.

Actions to Help a Person With a Bite or a Sting

Follow these first aid action steps for a person who has a bite or sting:

Actions to Help a Person With a Bite or a Sting
☐ Make sure the scene is safe for you and the person who has been stung or bitten.
☐ Get the first aid kit.
☐ Wear PPE.
☐ If the person was stung by a bee, scrape the stinger and venom sac away with something hard and dull that won't squeeze it—like the edge of a credit card or photo ID card.
☐ Wash the sting or bite area with running water and soap.
☐ Put a bag of ice and water wrapped in a towel over the area for up to 20 minutes.
☐ Watch the person for at least 30 minutes for signs of a severe allergic reaction. Be prepared to use the person's epinephrine pen if needed.

Allergic Reactions to Bee Stings

People who have had severe allergic reactions to an insect bite or sting usually have an epinephrine pen and know how to use it. They often wear medical identification jewelry.

Phone or send someone to phone 9-1-1 and get the first aid kit if the person develops a severe allergic reaction. Use the skills you learned earlier to help the person inject the epinephrine pen.

Poisonous Spider Bites and Scorpion Stings

The bite of nonpoisonous insects can cause mild signs of redness and itching at the bite area. However, the bite or sting of a poisonous spider or scorpion can cause a person to become ill.

Signs of poisonous spider bites and scorpion stings are

- Severe pain at the site of the bite or sting
- Muscle cramps
- Headache
- Fever
- Vomiting
- Breathing problems
- Seizures
- Lack of response

Actions to Help a Person Who Is Bitten or Stung by a Poisonous Spider or Scorpion

If you know that a person has been bitten or stung by a poisonous spider or scorpion or has any of these signs listed above after such a bite or sting, then follow these first aid action steps:

Actions to Help a Person Who Is Bitten or Stung by a Poisonous Spider or Scorpion
☐ Make sure the scene is safe for you and the person who was bitten or stung.
☐ Get the first aid kit.
☐ Wear PPE.
☐ Phone 9-1-1.
☐ Wash the bite or sting area with lots of running water and soap.
☐ Put a bag of ice and water wrapped in a towel on the bite or sting.

Tick Bites

Many ticks are harmless, but some carry serious diseases. They are found in wooded areas and attach themselves to exposed parts of the body.

If you find a tick, remove it as soon as possible. The longer the tick stays attached to a person, the greater the chance of catching a disease.

Actions to Help a Person Who Has a Tick Bite

The first aid actions for a tick bite begin with removing it from the person's body. Follow these first aid action steps for a person who has a tick bite:

Actions to Help a Person Who Has a Tick Bite
☐ Get the first aid kit.
☐ Wear PPE.
☐ Use tweezers to grab the tick by its mouth or head, as close to the skin as possible.
☐ Try to avoid pinching the tick.
☐ Lift the tick straight out. If you lift the tick until the person's skin tents and wait for several seconds, the tick may let go.
☐ Place the tick in a plastic bag in case the person needs to take it with him when getting medical care.
☐ Wash the bite area with running water and soap.
☐ If you are in an area where you know there is tick-borne illness, suggest that the person see a healthcare provider as soon as possible.

Marine Bites and Stings

Just as it's important to be aware of ticks and other insects and animals when you're in the wilderness, it's important to be aware of marine fish and animals when swimming in the ocean.

Bites and stings from jellyfish, stingray, or stonefish may cause pain, swelling, redness, or bleeding. Some marine bites and stings can be serious and even fatal if a person has a severe allergic reaction to the sting or the venom.

Actions to Help a Person Who Has a Marine Bite or Sting

Follow these first aid action steps for a marine bite or sting:

Actions to Help a Person Who Has a Marine Bite or Sting
☐ Make sure the scene is safe for you and the person who has been stung.
☐ Get the first aid kit.
☐ Wear PPE.
☐ Keep the injured person quiet and still.
☐ Wipe off stingers or tentacles with a gloved hand or towel.
☐ If the sting is from a jellyfish, rinse the injured area for at least 30 seconds with lots of vinegar. If vinegar is not available, use a baking soda and water solution instead.
☐ Put the part of the body that was stung in hot water. You may also have the person take a shower with water as hot as he can bear for at least 20 minutes or as long as pain persists.
☐ Phone 9-1-1 if • A person has been bitten or stung by a marine animal and has signs of a severe allergic reaction • A person was bitten or stung while in an area known to have poisonous marine animals
☐ For all bites and stings that break the skin, see a healthcare provider.

Heat-Related Emergencies

Dehydration

Working, training, or playing in extreme heat can be dangerous. If a person doesn't take the proper care, exposure to extremely hot environments can lead to life-threatening medical conditions.

Dehydration occurs when a person loses water or fluids through

- Heat exposure
- Too much exercise

- Vomiting, diarrhea, fever, or decreased fluid intake

If not responded to early, dehydration may lead to shock.

Signs of Dehydration

Signs of heat-related or environmental dehydration include

- Weakness
- Thirst or dry mouth
- Dizziness
- Confusion
- Less urination than usual

Actions to Take for Dehydration

If you suspect that a person is dehydrated, contact a healthcare provider right away. The best first aid for dehydration is prevention: make sure a person drinks and eats enough to stay hydrated.

Heat Cramps

Heat cramps are painful muscle spasms, most often occurring in the calves, arms, stomach muscles, and back.

Signs of Heat Cramps

Signs of heat cramps are

- Muscle cramps
- Sweating
- Headache

Heat cramps are a sign that heat-related problems may continue to get worse if the person doesn't take action.

Actions to Help a Person Who Has Heat Cramps

Follow these first aid action steps to help someone with heat cramps:

Actions to Help a Person Who Has Heat Cramps
☐ Get the first aid kit.
☐ Wear PPE.
☐ Have the person rest and cool off.
☐ Have the person drink something with sugar and electrolytes, such as a sports drink or juice, or water if these aren't available.
☐ If the person can tolerate it, apply a bag with ice and water wrapped in a towel to the cramping area for up to 20 minutes.

Heat Exhaustion

A milder condition, such as heat cramps, can quickly turn into heat exhaustion. That's why it's important to recognize and give first aid for heat-related emergencies early.

Signs of Heat Exhaustion

The signs of heat exhaustion are similar to those of heat stroke:

- Nausea
- Dizziness
- Vomiting
- Muscle cramps
- Feeling faint or fatigued
- Heavy sweating

Actions to Help a Person Who Has Heat Exhaustion

Follow these first aid action steps for heat exhaustion:

Actions to Help a Person Who Has Heat Exhaustion
☐ Get the first aid kit.
☐ Wear PPE.
☐ Phone 9-1-1.
☐ Have the person lie down in a cool place.
☐ Remove as much of the person's clothing as possible.
☐ Cool the person with a cool water spray. If a cool water spray is not available, place cool, damp cloths on the neck, armpits, and groin.
☐ If the person is responsive and can drink, have the person drink something with sugar and electrolytes, such as a sports drink or juice, or water if these aren't available.

Heat Stroke

Heat-related conditions can progress quickly if not recognized and treated. Heat stroke is a dangerous condition that is life threatening.

It's important to begin cooling a person who might have heat stroke immediately—every minute counts. If you can't immerse the person in water, try to cool him with a cool water spray.

If the person starts behaving normally again, stop cooling him. If you keep cooling the person, it could actually lead to low body temperature.

Signs of Heat Stroke

Signs of heat stroke are

- Confusion
- Feeling faint or fatigued
- Dizziness
- Fainting
- Nausea or vomiting
- Muscle cramps
- Seizure

Actions to Help a Person Who Has Heat Stroke

Follow these first aid action steps to help someone with heat stroke:

Actions to Help a Person Who Has Heat Stroke
☐ Phone 9-1-1.
☐ Put the person in cool water up to his neck if possible, or spray him with cool water.
☐ If the person becomes unresponsive and is not breathing normally or only gasping, give CPR.

Cold-Related Emergencies

Frostbite

Frostbite typically occurs outside in cold weather. But it can also occur inside or in a workplace if people are exposed to extremely cold materials, such as cold gases, without wearing gloves.

Signs of Frostbite

Frostbite affects parts of the body that are exposed to the cold, such as the fingers, toes, nose, and ears.

The signs of frostbite are the following:

- The skin over the frostbitten area is white, waxy, or grayish-yellow.
- The frostbitten area is cold and numb.
- The frostbitten area is hard, and the skin doesn't move when you push it.

Actions to Help a Person Who Has Frostbite

Follow these first aid action steps for frostbite:

Actions to Help a Person Who Has Frostbite
☐ Make sure the scene is safe for you and the person with frostbite.
☐ Move the person to a warm place.
☐ Get the first aid kit.
☐ Wear PPE.
☐ Phone 9-1-1.
☐ Remove wet or tight clothing and pat the body dry.
☐ Put dry clothes on the person and cover him with a blanket.
☐ Remove tight rings or any bracelets from the frostbitten part.

Caution

These are things you *should not do* for frostbite:

- Do not try to thaw the frozen part if you think there may be a chance of the body refreezing before the person can get to medical care.
- Do not rub the frostbitten area. Rubbing it may cause damage. If you need to touch the area, do so gently.

Low Body Temperature (Hypothermia)

Hypothermia is another name for low body temperature. Staying too long in a cold, pouring rain or other wet and cold conditions can lead to hypothermia. A person can develop low body temperature even when the outside temperature is above freezing.

When hypothermia occurs, it can cause serious problems or even death.

Signs of Low Body Temperature

The signs of low body temperature may include

- Skin that's cool to the touch
- Shivering, which stops when the body temperature is very low
- Confusion
- Personality change
- Sleepiness and the person's lack of concern about his condition
- Stiff, rigid muscles while the skin becomes ice-cold and blue

As the person's body temperature continues to drop, it may be hard to tell if the person is breathing. The person may become unresponsive and even appear to be dead.

Actions to Help a Person Who Has Hypothermia

Follow these first aid action steps for a person with low body temperature:

Actions to Help a Person Who Has Hypothermia
☐ Make sure the scene is safe for you and the person who has hypothermia.
☐ Get the person out of the cold.
☐ Remove wet clothing, pat the person dry, and cover with a blanket.
☐ Get the first aid kit and AED.
☐ Phone 9-1-1.
☐ Put dry clothes on the person. • Cover the body and head, but not the face, with blankets, towels, or even newspapers.
☐ Remain with the person until someone with more advanced training arrives and takes over.
☐ If the person becomes unresponsive and is not breathing normally or only gasping, give CPR.

Poison Emergencies

A poison is anything that someone swallows or breathes or that gets into the eyes or on the skin and that causes sickness or death. Many products can poison people.

Poison Control Hotline

The phone number for the poison control center should be in the first aid kit or prominently displayed in the areas where chemicals are used.

Contact your local poison center by phoning the American Association of Poison Control Centers (Poison Control) at

1-800-222-1222

Questions the Poison Control Center Dispatcher May Ask

When you call the Poison Control Center, the dispatcher may ask for the following information:

- What is the name of the poison?
- Can you describe it if you can't name it?
- How much poison did the person touch, breathe, or swallow?
- How old is the person?
- How much does the person weigh?
- When did the poisoning happen?
- How is the person feeling or acting now?

Actions to Take for Scene Safety in a Poison Emergency

If someone has been exposed to a poison, first make sure the scene is safe. For example, you may need to look for spills of liquids or powders that might be poison.

Follow these actions steps before doing anything else:

Actions to Take for Scene Safety in a Poison Emergency
☐ Make sure the scene is safe for you and the ill or injured person before you approach.
☐ Look for signs that warn you that poisons are nearby (Figure 29).
☐ Look for spilled or leaking containers.
☐ If the scene seems unsafe, do not approach. Tell everyone to move away.
☐ Stay out of the scene if you see multiple people who may have been poisoned.
☐ If the scene is safe, get the first aid kit and AED.
☐ Phone 9-1-1.
☐ Tell the dispatcher the name of the poison if you know it. Some dispatchers may connect you to a poison control center. Give only those antidotes that the poison control center or dispatcher tells you to. The first aid instructions on the poison itself can be helpful but may be incomplete.

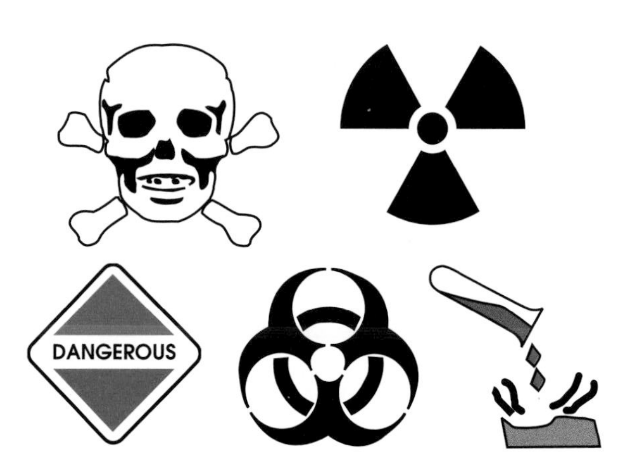

Figure 29. Look for symbols of poisons, such as these.

Safety Data Sheet

Some places have a safety data sheet, or SDS, that provides a description of how a specific chemical or poison can be harmful. It may have first aid recommendations as well.

Actions to Help a Person Who Has Poison on the Skin or in the Eyes

Follow these first aid action steps to remove poison from a person's skin or eyes.

Actions to Help a Person Who Has Poison on the Skin or in the Eyes
☐ Make sure the scene is safe for you and the ill or injured person by following the "Actions to Take for Scene Safety in a Poison Emergency" section.
☐ If you approach the scene, wear PPE.
☐ Move the person from the scene of the poison if you can, and help the person move to an area with fresh air.
☐ As quickly and as safely as you can, wash or remove the poison from the person's skin and clothing. Help the person to a faucet, safety shower, or eyewash station.
☐ Remove clothing and jewelry from any part of the body touched by the poison. Use a gloved hand to brush off any dry powder or solid substance from the person's skin (Figure 30).
☐ Run lots of water over the affected area until someone with more advanced training arrives and takes over.

(continued)

(continued)

Actions to Help a Person Who Has Poison on the Skin or in the Eyes
☐ If an eye is affected, ask the person to blink as much as possible while rinsing the eyes. If only one eye is affected, make sure the eye with the poison in it is the lower eye so that you don't rinse the poison into the unaffected eye.
☐ Give CPR if the person becomes unresponsive and isn't breathing normally or is only gasping. Use a mask for providing breaths. This is especially important if the poison has contaminated the person's lips or mouth.

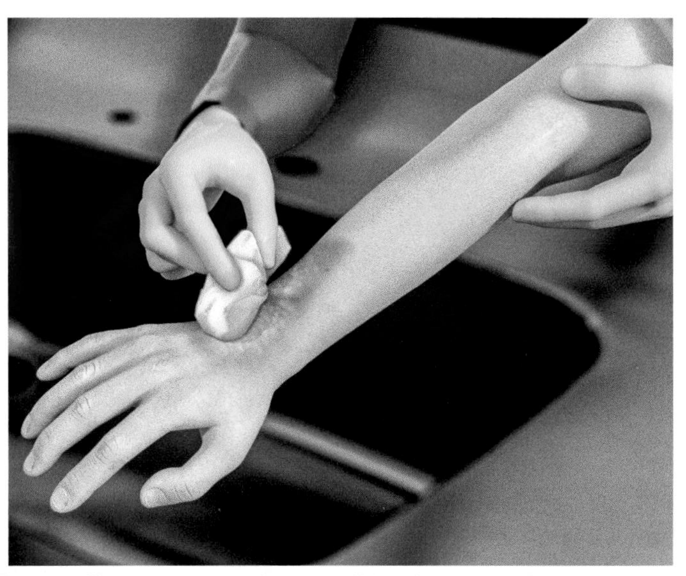

Figure 30. Brush off any dry powder or solid substances from the person's skin with your gloved hand.

Environmental Emergencies: Review Questions

Question	Your Notes
1. Someone who has been bitten by an insect or bee may have a severe allergic reaction and should be watched for at least _____ minutes. a. 10 b. 20 c. 30 d. 60	
2. When someone has a bite, be sure to wash the bite area with a lot of soap and water. True False	
3. Heat stroke is a life-threatening condition. True False	
4. Remove ticks _____. a. with a hot matchstick b. with lots of alcohol on the skin c. by using tweezers d. with your hands	
5. Being confused may be a symptom of heat stroke and low body temperature. True False	
6. If you give CPR to someone who has been poisoned, it is important to use a mask, if possible, to give breaths. True False	

Answers: **1.** c, **2.** True, **3.** True, **4.** c, **5.** True, **6.** True

Part 5: Preventing Illness and Injury

Preventing illness and injury is an important part of providing first aid.

Watching and being able to see an accident coming and taking precautions against someone getting ill are all part of your role as a first aid rescuer.

Review Often to Be Prepared to Act

Review your Student Workbook and the Quick Reference Guides often to keep your knowledge and skills fresh.

Even if you don't remember all the steps exactly, it is important for you to try. Any help, even if it isn't perfect, is better than no help at all.

More than anything, we want you to act in an emergency and have the confidence to do so. Recognizing that something is wrong and getting help on the way is one of the most important things you can do.

Laws to Protect the Rescuer

If you have questions regarding whether or not it's legal to provide someone first aid, all states have Good Samaritan laws. These laws protect anyone who provides first aid. They differ from state to state, so be sure to refer to the Good Samaritan laws in your local area.

More Information and Training

Contact the American Heart Association if you want more information on first aid, CPR, or AED training. You can visit **www.heart.org/cpr** or call 1-877-AHA-4CPR (877-242-4277) to find a class near you.

Thank You

Thank you for completing this section of the Heartsaver First Aid CPR AED Course.

Remember, first aid can be initiated by anyone in any situation. As a first aid rescuer, you can help save a life, reduce suffering, and prevent further illness or injury, as well as help someone with an illness or injury get better faster.

Part 6: First Aid Resources

Sample First Aid Kit

Below is a sample list of contents for a first aid kit. This kit follows the standard of the Occupational Safety and Health Administration (OSHA). Different workplaces may have different requirements. The American National Standards Institute (ANSI) and the International Safety Equipment Association (ISEA) also have a standard for contents of first aid kits, available at **ansi.org**.

The contents listed below are enough for small workplaces with about 2 or 3 employees. Larger workplaces need more first aid kits or extra supplies.

1. Gauze pads (at least 4 × 4 inches)
2. Two large gauze pads (at least 8 × 10 inches)
3. Box of adhesive bandages
4. One package of gauze roller bandage, at least 2 inches wide
5. Two triangular bandages
6. Wound cleaning agent, such as sealed, moistened towelettes
7. Scissors
8. At least 1 blanket
9. Tweezers
10. Adhesive tape
11. Latex gloves
12. Resuscitation equipment, such as a pocket mask
13. Two elastic wraps
14. Splint
15. Directions for requesting emergency assistance (including list of important local emergency telephone numbers, such as police, fire department, EMS, and poison control center*)
16. Heartsaver First Aid Quick Reference Guide*

*Items marked with an asterisk are in addition to those listed in the OSHA 1910.266 App A standard.

CPR and AED

Although much is being done to prevent death from heart problems, sudden cardiac arrest is still one of the leading causes of death in the United States. About 70% of the arrests that occur outside of the hospital happen at home.

In this part, you will learn skills that will help you to recognize cardiac arrest, get emergency care on the way quickly, and help the person until more advanced care arrives to take over.

Life Is Why

High-Quality CPR Is Why

Early recognition and CPR are crucial for survival from cardiac arrest. By learning high-quality CPR, you'll have the knowledge and skills that may help save a life.

CPR AED Course Objectives

At the end of the CPR AED portion of this course, you will be able to

- Describe how high-quality CPR improves survival
- Explain the concepts of the Chain of Survival
- Recognize when someone needs CPR
- Perform high-quality CPR for an adult
- Describe how to perform CPR with help from others
- Give effective breaths by using mouth-to-mouth or a mask for all age groups
- Demonstrate how to use an AED on an adult
- Perform high-quality CPR for a child
- Demonstrate how to use an AED on a child
- Perform high-quality CPR for an infant
- Describe when and how to help a choking adult or child
- Demonstrate how to help a choking infant

CPR and AED Use for Adults

What You Will Learn

In this section, you will learn when CPR is needed, how to give CPR to an adult, and how to use an AED.

Adult Chain of Survival

The AHA adult Chain of Survival (Figure 31) shows the most important actions needed to treat adults who have cardiac arrests outside of a hospital.

In this part, you will learn about the first 3 links of the chain. The fourth and fifth links are advanced care provided by emergency responders and hospital providers who will take over care.

Link	Action
First link	Immediately recognize the emergency and phone 9-1-1.
Second link	Perform early CPR with an emphasis on chest compressions.
Third link	Use an AED immediately (as soon as it is available).

Remember that seconds count when someone has a cardiac arrest. Wherever you are, take action. The adult Chain of Survival starts with you!

Figure 31. The AHA adult Chain of Survival for cardiac arrests that occur outside of a hospital.

Topics Covered

- Assess and Phone 9-1-1
- Perform High-Quality CPR
- Use an AED
- Putting It All Together: Adult High-Quality CPR AED Summary

When you encounter an adult who may have had a cardiac arrest, take the following steps to assess the emergency and get help:

- Make sure the scene is safe.
- Tap and shout (check for responsiveness).
- Shout for help.
- Phone 9-1-1 and get an AED.
- Check for normal breathing.

Depending on the particular circumstance and the resources you have available, you may be able to perform some of these actions at the same time. You might, for example, phone 9-1-1 with your cell phone on speaker mode while checking for breathing.

Make Sure the Scene Is Safe

Before you assess the person, make sure the scene is safe. Look for anything nearby that might hurt you. You can't help if you get hurt too.

Some places that may be unsafe are

- A busy street or parking lot
- An area where power lines are down
- A room with poisonous fumes

As you give care, be aware if anything changes and makes it unsafe for you or the person needing help.

Tap and Shout (Check for Responsiveness)

Tap and shout to check if the person is responsive or unresponsive (Figure 32).

Lean over the person or kneel at his side. Tap his shoulders and ask if he is OK.

If	Then
The person moves, speaks, blinks, or otherwise reacts when you tap him.	He is *responsive*. Ask the person if he needs help.
The person doesn't move, speak, blink, or otherwise react when you tap him.	He is *unresponsive*. Shout for help so that if others are nearby, they can help you.

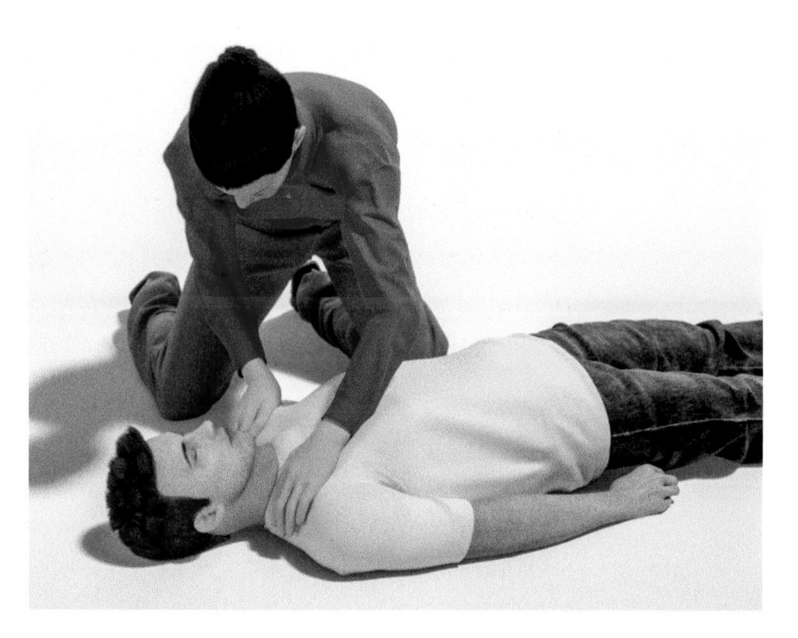

Figure 32. Tap and shout (check for responsiveness).

Shout for Help

In an emergency, the sooner you realize that there's a problem and get additional help, the better it is for the person with a cardiac arrest. When more people are helping, you are able to provide better care to the person.

If the person is unresponsive, shout for help (Figure 33).

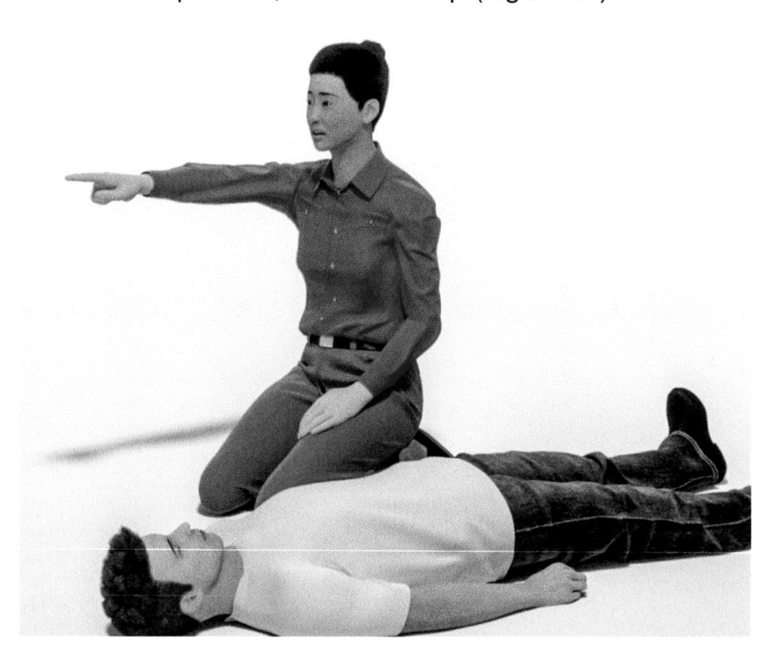

Figure 33. Shout for help.

Phone 9-1-1 and Get an AED

If someone comes to help and a cell phone is available

Ask the person to phone 9-1-1 and get an AED. Say, "You—phone 9-1-1 and get an AED." Ask that the phone be placed on speaker mode so that you can hear the dispatcher's instructions.

If someone comes to help and a cell phone is not available

Ask the person to go phone 9-1-1 and get an AED while you continue providing emergency care.

If you are alone and have a cell phone or nearby phone

If no one comes to help, phone 9-1-1. Put the phone on speaker mode so that you can hear the dispatcher's instructions while you continue providing emergency care. If an AED is needed, you will have to go get it yourself.

If you are alone and don't have a cell phone

Leave the person to go phone 9-1-1 and get an AED. Return and continue providing emergency care.

Follow the Dispatcher's Instructions

Stay on the phone until the 9-1-1 dispatcher tells you to hang up. Answering the dispatcher's questions will not delay the arrival of help.

The dispatcher will ask you about the emergency—where you are and what has happened. Dispatchers can provide instructions that will help you, such as telling you how to provide CPR, use an AED, or give first aid.

That's why it's important to put the phone on speaker mode after phoning 9-1-1 so that the dispatcher and the person providing CPR can speak to each other.

Check for Normal Breathing

If the person is unresponsive, check for normal breathing (Figure 34).

Scan the chest from head to chest repeatedly for at least 5 seconds (but no more than 10 seconds) looking for chest rise and fall. If the person is not breathing normally or is only gasping, he needs CPR. (See "Heartsaver First Aid CPR AED Terms and Concepts" for more information on gasping.)

If	Then
The person is unresponsive and is breathing normally.	• This person does not need CPR. • Roll him onto his side (if you don't think he has a neck or back injury). This will help keep the airway clear in the event the person vomits. • Stay with the person until advanced help arrives.
The person is unresponsive and not breathing normally or is only gasping.	• This person needs CPR. • Make sure the person is lying on his back on a firm, flat surface. • Begin CPR.

Remember	Unresponsive + No normal breathing or only gasping = **Provide CPR**

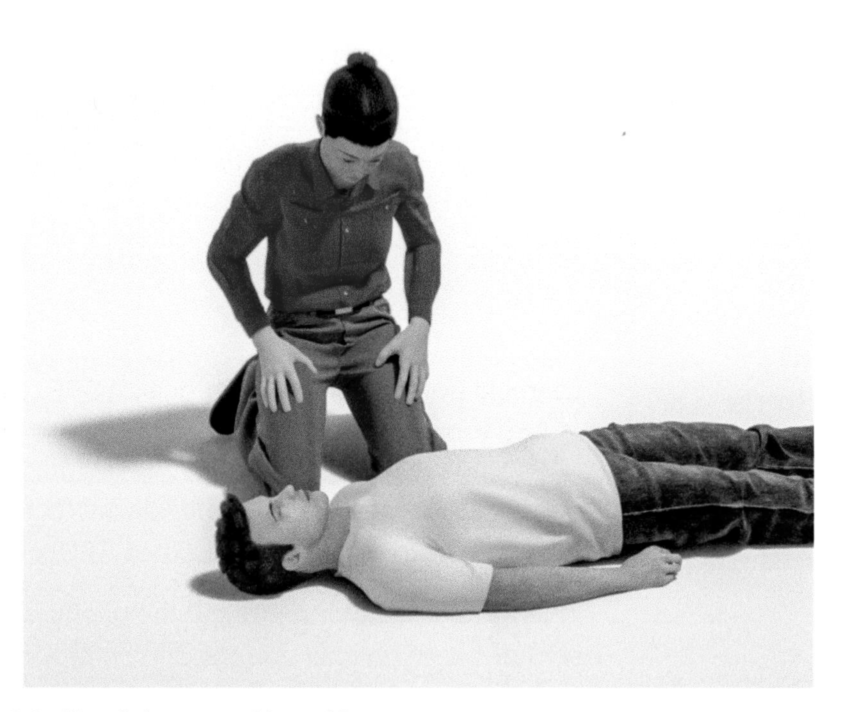

Figure 34. Check for normal breathing.

What to Do If You Are Not Sure

If you think someone needs CPR but you aren't sure, provide CPR because you may save a life. CPR is not likely to cause harm if the person is not in cardiac arrest.

It's better to give CPR to someone who doesn't need it than not to give it to someone who does need it.

Summary

Here is a summary of how to assess the emergency and get help when you encounter an ill or injured adult:

Assess and Phone 9-1-1
☐ Make sure the scene is safe.
• Tap and shout (check for responsiveness). • If the person is *responsive,* ask him if he needs help. • If the person is *unresponsive,* go to the next step.
☐ Shout for help.

(continued)

(continued)

☐ Phone 9-1-1 and get an AED.

- Phone or send someone to phone 9-1-1 and get an AED.
- If you're alone and have a cell phone or a nearby phone, put it on speaker mode and phone 9-1-1.

☐ Check for breathing.

- If the person is breathing normally, stay with the person until advanced help arrives.
- If the person is *not* breathing normally or only gasping, begin CPR and use an AED. See "Perform High-Quality CPR."

Perform High-Quality CPR

Learning how to perform high-quality CPR is important. The better the CPR skills are performed, the better the chances of survival.

Life Is Why

Saving Lives Is Why

Sudden cardiac arrest remains a leading cause of death, so the American Heart Association trains millions of people each year to help save lives both in and out of the hospital.

CPR Skills

CPR has 2 main skills:

- Providing compressions
- Giving breaths

You will learn how to perform these skills for an adult in cardiac arrest in this section.

Provide Compressions

A compression is the act of pushing hard and fast on the chest. When you push on the chest, you pump blood to the brain and heart.

To provide high-quality compressions, make sure that you

- Provide compressions that are deep enough
- Provide compressions that are fast enough
- Let the chest come back up to its normal position after each compression
- Try not to interrupt compressions for more than 10 seconds, even when you give breaths

Compression depth is an important part of providing high-quality compressions. You need to push hard enough to pump blood through the body. It's better to push too hard than not hard enough. People are often afraid of causing a person injury by providing compressions, but injury is unlikely.

Compression Technique

Here is how to provide compressions for an adult during CPR (Figure 35):

How to Provide Compressions for an Adult During CPR
☐ Make sure the person is lying on his back on a firm, flat surface.
☐ Quickly move clothes out of the way.
☐ Put the heel of one hand on the center of the chest (over the lower half of the breastbone). Put your other hand on top of the first hand (Figure 35).
☐ Push straight down at least 2 inches.
☐ Push at a rate of 100 to 120 compressions per minute. Count the compressions out loud.
☐ Let the chest come back up to its normal position after each compression.
☐ Try not to interrupt compressions for more than 10 seconds, even when you give breaths.

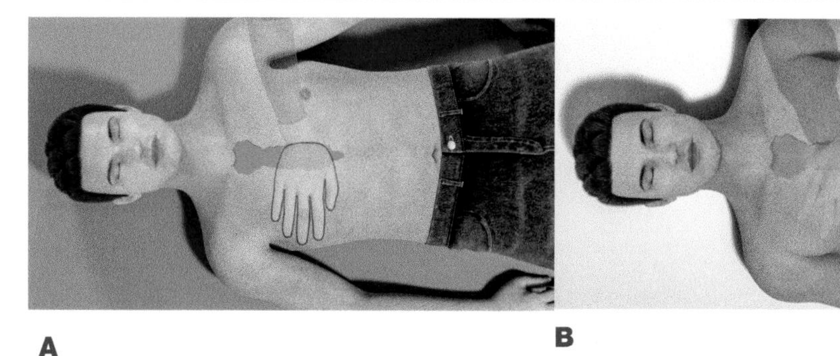

Figure 35. Compressions. **A,** Put the heel of one hand on the center of the chest (lower half of the breastbone). **B,** Put the other hand on top of the first hand.

Switch Rescuers to Avoid Fatigue

Performing chest compressions correctly is hard work. The more tired you become, the less effective your compressions will be.

If someone else knows CPR, you can take turns providing CPR (Figure 36). Switch rescuers about every 2 minutes, or sooner if you get tired. Move quickly to keep any pauses in compressions as short as possible.

Remind other rescuers to perform high-quality CPR as described in the box labeled "How to Provide Compressions for an Adult During CPR."

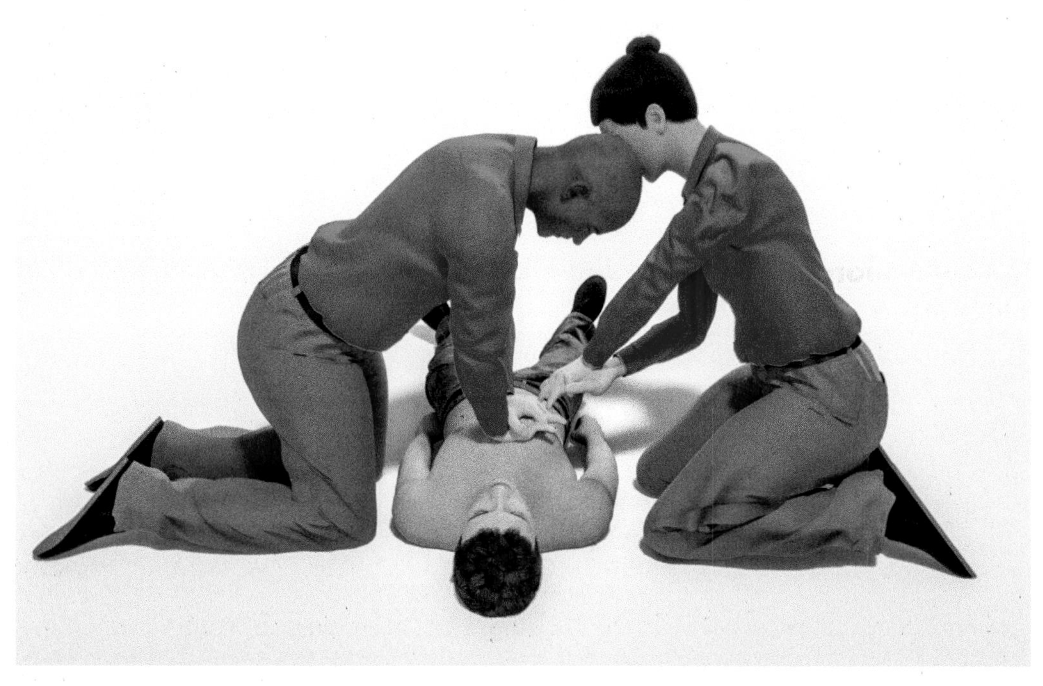

Figure 36. Switch rescuers about every 2 minutes to avoid fatigue.

Give Breaths

The second skill of CPR is giving breaths. After each set of 30 compressions, you will need to give 2 breaths. Breaths may be given with or without a barrier device, such as a pocket mask or face shield.

When you give breaths, the breaths need to make the chest rise visibly. When you can see the chest rise, you know you have delivered an effective breath.

Open the Airway

Before giving breaths, open the airway (Figure 37). This lifts the tongue from the back of the throat to make sure your breaths get air into the lungs.

Follow these steps to open the airway:

How to Open the Airway
☐ Put one hand on the forehead and the fingers of your other hand on the bony part of the chin (Figure 37).
☐ Tilt the head back and lift the chin.

Avoid pressing into the soft part of the neck or under the chin because this might block the airway.

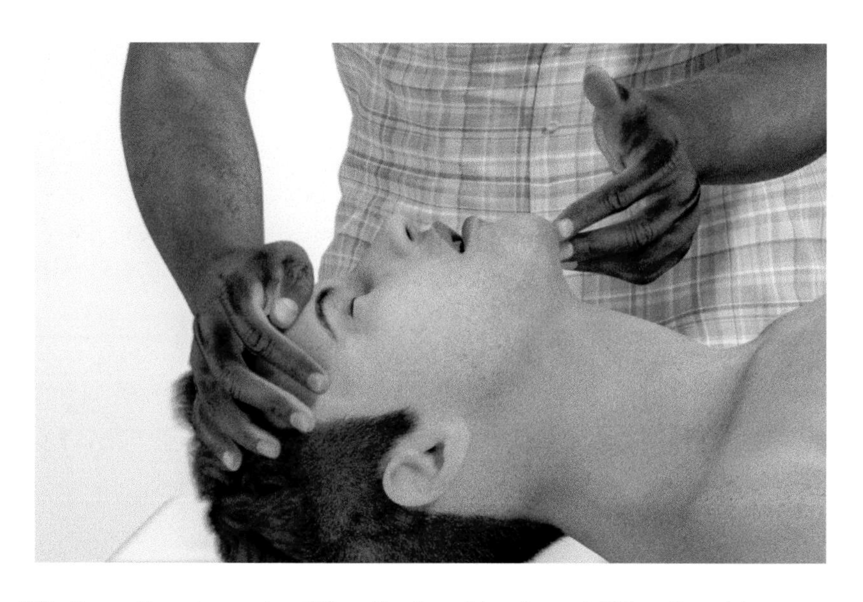

Figure 37. Open the airway by tilting the head back and lifting the chin.

Give Breaths Without a Pocket Mask

If you choose to give someone breaths without a barrier device, it is usually quite safe because there is very little chance that you will catch a disease.

Follow these steps to give breaths without a pocket mask or face shield (Figure 38).

How to Give Breaths (Without a Pocket Mask)
☐ While holding the airway open, pinch the nose closed with your thumb and forefinger.
☐ Take a normal breath. Cover the person's mouth with your mouth.
☐ Give 2 breaths (blow for 1 second for each). Watch for the chest to begin to rise as you give each breath.
☐ Try not to interrupt compressions for more than 10 seconds.

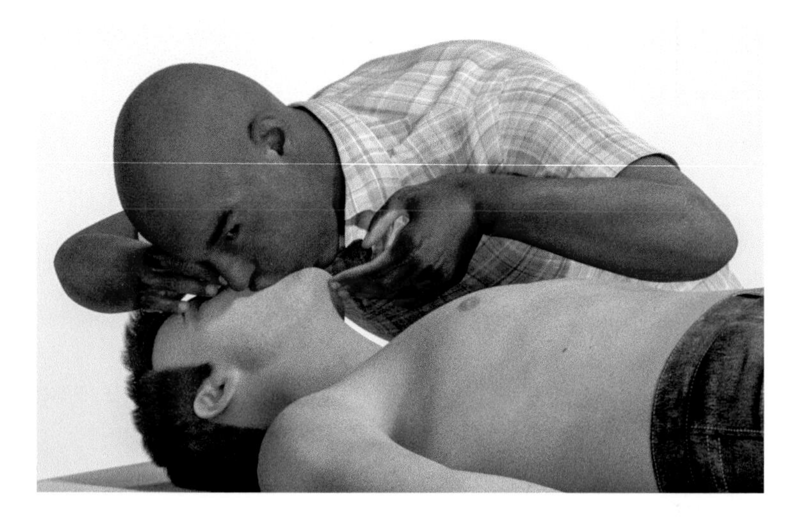

Figure 38. Give breaths.

What to Do If the Chest Doesn't Rise

It takes a little practice to give breaths correctly. If you give someone a breath and the chest doesn't rise, do the following:

- Allow the head to go back to its normal position.
- Open the airway again by tilting the head back and lifting the chin.
- Then, give another breath. Make sure the chest rises.

Minimize Interruptions in Chest Compressions

If you have been unable to give 2 effective breaths in 10 seconds, go back to pushing hard and fast on the chest. Try to give breaths again after every 30 compressions.

Don't interrupt compressions for more than 10 seconds.

Use a Pocket Mask

You may give breaths with or without a barrier device, such as a pocket mask. Barrier devices are made of plastic and fit over the person's mouth and nose (Figure 39). They protect the rescuer from blood, vomit, or disease. Your instructor may discuss other types of barrier devices, like face shields, which can be used when giving breaths.

If you're in the workplace, your employer may provide personal protective equipment, including pocket masks or face shields, for use during CPR.

There are many different kinds of pocket masks as well as different sizes for adults, children, and infants. So, make sure you're using the right size. You may need to put a pocket mask together before you use it.

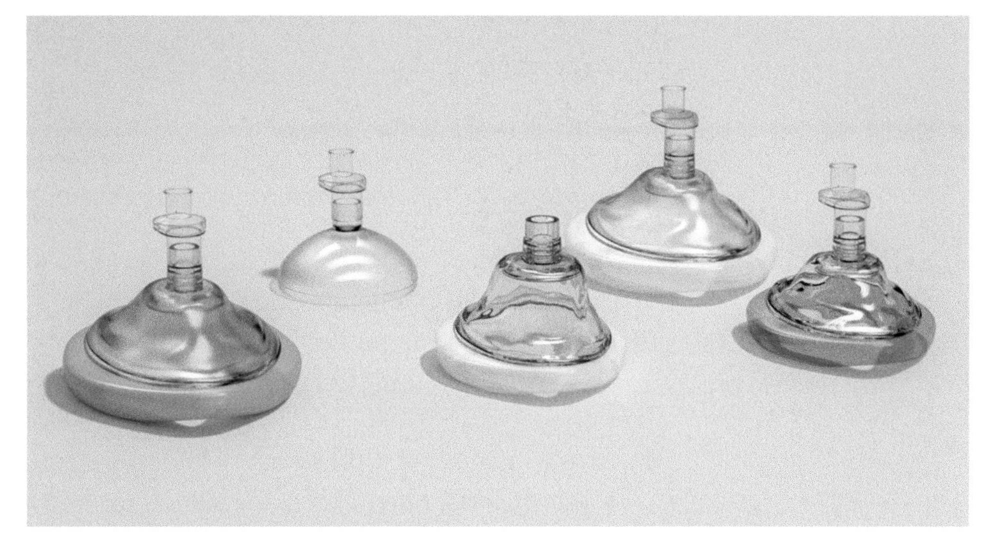

Figure 39. Some people use a pocket mask when giving breaths.

Give Breaths With a Pocket Mask

Follow these steps to give breaths with a pocket mask (Figure 40):

How to Give Breaths With a Pocket Mask
☐ Put the mask over the person's mouth and nose. • If the mask has a pointed end, put the narrow end of the mask on the bridge of the nose; position the wide end so that it covers the mouth.
☐ Tilt the head and lift the chin while pressing the mask against the person's face. It is important to make an airtight seal between the person's face and the mask while you lift the chin to keep the airway open.
☐ Give 2 breaths (blow for 1 second for each). Watch for the chest to begin to rise as you give each breath.
☐ Try not to interrupt compressions for more than 10 seconds.

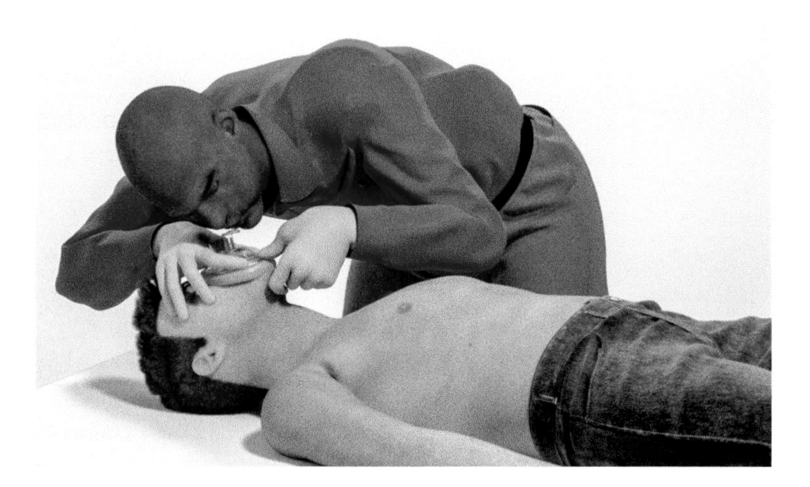

Figure 40. Giving breaths with a pocket mask.

Give Sets of 30 Compressions and 2 Breaths

When providing CPR, give sets of 30 compressions and 2 breaths.

How to Give Sets of Compressions and Breaths to an Adult
☐ Make sure the person is lying on his back on a firm, flat surface.
☐ Quickly move clothes out of the way.
☐ Give 30 chest compressions. • Put the heel of one hand on the center of the chest (over the lower half of the breastbone). Put your other hand on top of the first hand. • Push straight down at least 2 inches. • Push at a rate of 100 to 120 compressions per minute. Count the compressions out loud. • Let the chest come back up to its normal position after each compression.

(continued)

(continued)

- ☐ After 30 compressions, give 2 breaths.
  - Open the airway and give 2 breaths (blow for 1 second for each). Watch for the chest to begin to rise as you give each breath.
  - Try not to interrupt compressions for more than 10 seconds.

Use an AED

CPR combined with using an AED provides the best chance of saving a life. If possible, use an AED every time you provide CPR.

AEDs are safe, accurate, and easy to use. Once you turn on the AED, follow the prompts. The AED will analyze if the person needs a shock and will automatically give one or tell you when to give one.

Turn on the AED

To use an AED, turn it on by either pushing the "on" button or lifting the lid (Figure 41). Once you turn on the AED, you will hear prompts, which will tell you everything you need to do.

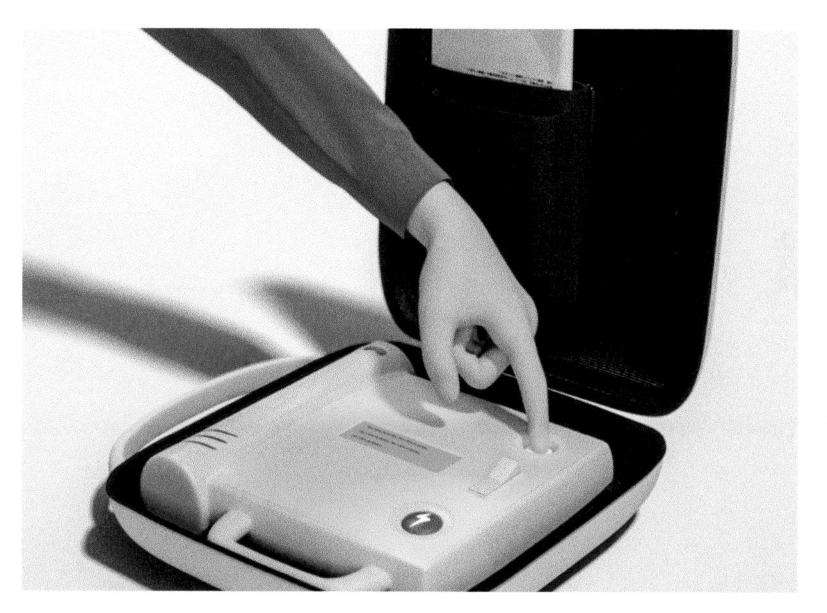

Figure 41. Turning on the AED.

Attach the Pads

AEDs may have adult and child pads. Make sure you use the adult pads for anyone 8 years of age or older. Before you place the pads, quickly scan the person to see if there are any special situations that might require additional steps. See "Special Situations" below.

Peel away the backing from the pads. Following the pictures on the pads, attach them to the person's bare chest (Figure 42).

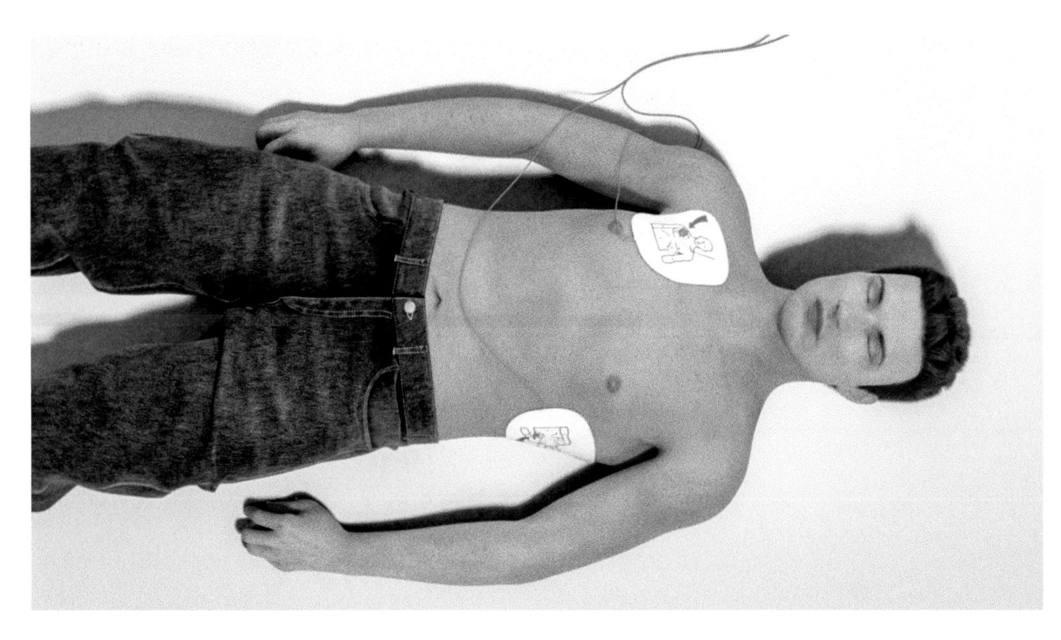

Figure 42. Place pads on an adult by following the pictures on the pads.

Clear the Person if a Shock Is Advised

Let the AED analyze the heart rhythm. If the AED advises a shock, it will tell you to stay clear of the person. If so, then loudly state, "Clear." Make sure that no one is touching the person just before you push the "shock" button (Figure 43).

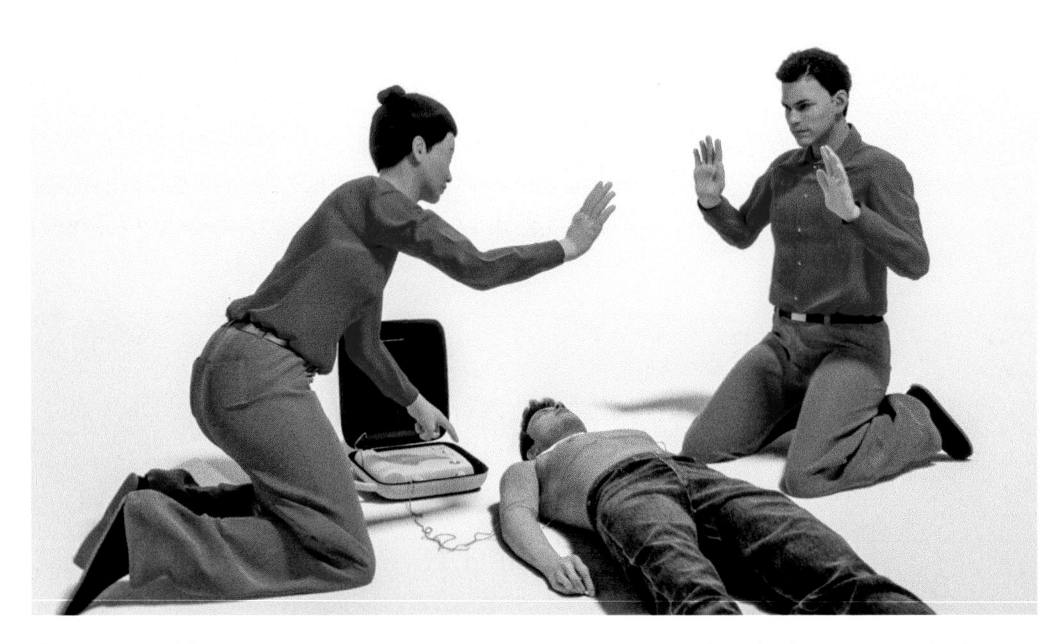

Figure 43. Make sure that no one is touching the person just before you push the "shock" button.

Steps for Using an AED for an Adult

Use the AED as soon as it is available. Here are the steps for using an AED for an adult:

How to Use an AED for an Adult
☐ Turn the AED on and follow the prompts. • Turn it on by pushing the "on" button or lifting the lid (Figure 41). • Follow the prompts, which will tell you everything you need to do.
☐ Attach the adult pads. • Use the adult pads for anyone 8 years of age and older. • Peel away the backing from the pads. • Following the pictures on the pads, attach them to the person's bare chest (Figure 42).
☐ Let the AED analyze. • Loudly state, "Clear," and make sure that no one is touching the person. • The AED will analyze the heart rhythm. • If a shock is not needed, resume CPR.
☐ Deliver a shock if needed (Figure 43). • Loudly state, "Clear," and make sure that no one is touching the person. • Push the "shock" button. • Immediately resume CPR.

Special Situations

There are some special situations that you may need to consider before placing AED pads. Quickly scan the person to see if he has any of the following *before* applying the pads:

If the victim...	Then
Has hair on the chest that may prevent pads from sticking	• Quickly shave the area where you will place the pads using the razor from the AED carrying case. *or* • Remove the hair by using a second set of AED pads (if available). – Apply the pads and press them down firmly. – Rip the pads off forcefully to remove the chest hair. – Reapply a new set of pads to the bare skin.
Is lying in water	• Quickly move the victim to a dry area.

(continued)

(continued)

Is lying on snow or in a small puddle	• You may use the AED (the chest doesn't have to be completely dry). • If the chest is covered with water or sweat, quickly wipe it before attaching the pads.
Has water on the chest	• Quickly wipe the chest dry before attaching the pads.
Has an implanted defibrillator or pacemaker	• Don't put the AED pad directly over the implanted device. • Follow the normal steps for operating an AED.
Has a medicine patch where you need to place an AED pad	• Don't put the AED pad directly over a medicine patch. • Use protective gloves. • Remove the medicated patch. • Wipe the area clean. • Attach the AED pads.

Continue Providing CPR and Using the AED

As soon as the AED gives the shock, immediately resume chest compressions. Continue to follow the AED prompts, which will guide the rescue.

Provide CPR and use the AED until

- Someone else arrives who can take turns providing CPR with you
- The person begins to move, speak, blink, or otherwise react
- Someone with more advanced training arrives

Putting It All Together: Adult High-Quality CPR AED Summary

Compressions are very important to deliver blood flow and are the core of CPR. Try not to interrupt chest compressions for more than 10 seconds when you give breaths.

Assess and Phone 9-1-1
☐ Make sure the scene is safe.
☐ Tap and shout (check for responsiveness). • If the person is *responsive,* ask him if he needs help. • If the person is *unresponsive,* go to the next step.
☐ Shout for help.

(continued)

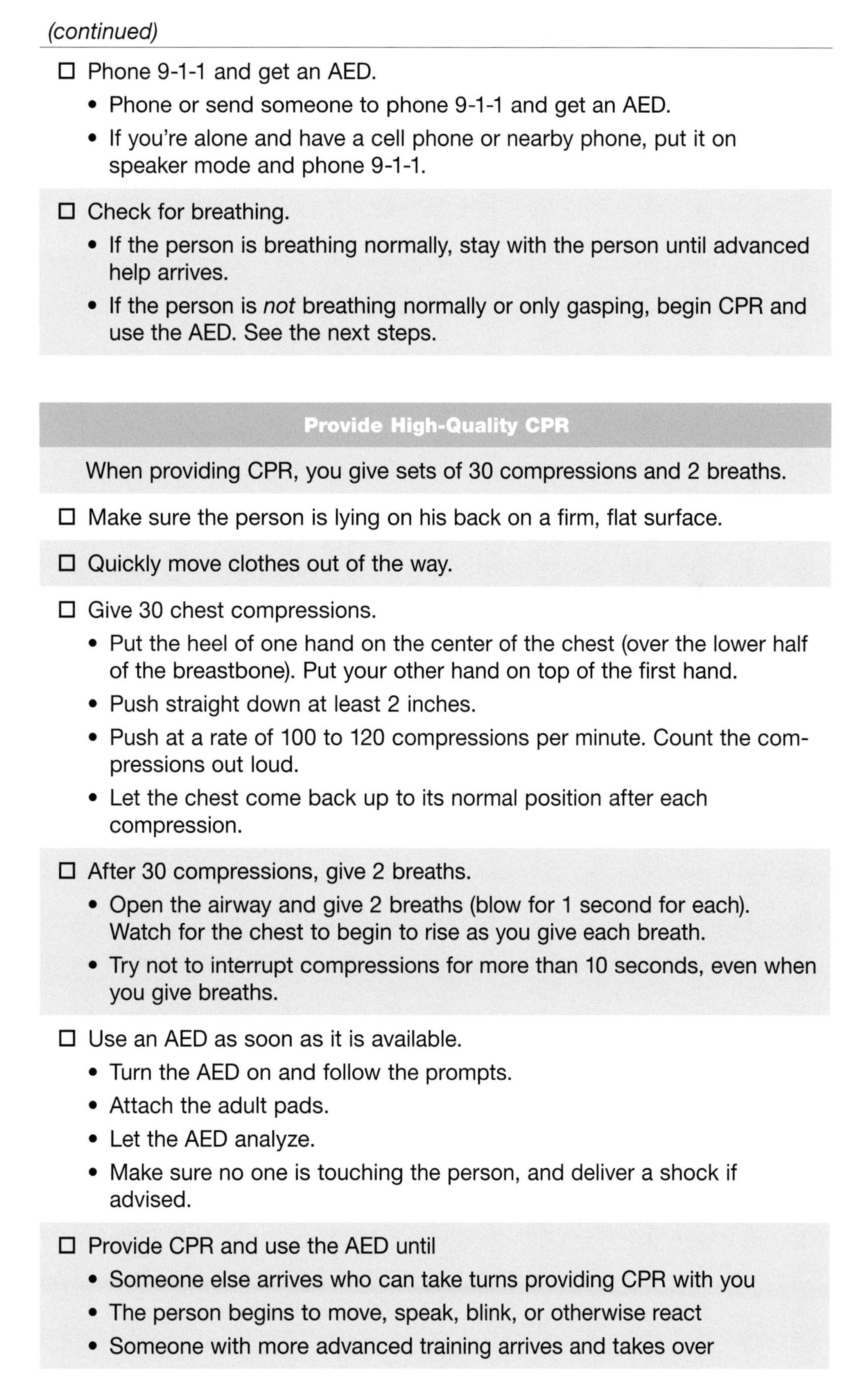

(continued)

- ☐ Phone 9-1-1 and get an AED.
  - Phone or send someone to phone 9-1-1 and get an AED.
  - If you're alone and have a cell phone or nearby phone, put it on speaker mode and phone 9-1-1.
- ☐ Check for breathing.
  - If the person is breathing normally, stay with the person until advanced help arrives.
  - If the person is *not* breathing normally or only gasping, begin CPR and use the AED. See the next steps.

Provide High-Quality CPR

When providing CPR, you give sets of 30 compressions and 2 breaths.

- ☐ Make sure the person is lying on his back on a firm, flat surface.
- ☐ Quickly move clothes out of the way.
- ☐ Give 30 chest compressions.
  - Put the heel of one hand on the center of the chest (over the lower half of the breastbone). Put your other hand on top of the first hand.
  - Push straight down at least 2 inches.
  - Push at a rate of 100 to 120 compressions per minute. Count the compressions out loud.
  - Let the chest come back up to its normal position after each compression.
- ☐ After 30 compressions, give 2 breaths.
  - Open the airway and give 2 breaths (blow for 1 second for each). Watch for the chest to begin to rise as you give each breath.
  - Try not to interrupt compressions for more than 10 seconds, even when you give breaths.
- ☐ Use an AED as soon as it is available.
  - Turn the AED on and follow the prompts.
  - Attach the adult pads.
  - Let the AED analyze.
  - Make sure no one is touching the person, and deliver a shock if advised.
- ☐ Provide CPR and use the AED until
  - Someone else arrives who can take turns providing CPR with you
  - The person begins to move, speak, blink, or otherwise react
  - Someone with more advanced training arrives and takes over

In the United States, drug overdoses now kill more adults each year than motor vehicle crashes do. Many overdoses are from prescription drugs. Opioids are prescription drugs used for pain relief but are often abused. Common opioids are morphine and hydrocodone. Heroin is an example of an opioid that is illegal in the United States.

Naloxone Reverses Effects of Opioids

Naloxone is a drug that reverses the effects of opioids. It is safe and effective. Emergency responders have used naloxone for many years.

Family members or caregivers of known opioid users may have naloxone close by to use in case of an opioid overdose.

If you know someone who has a prescription for naloxone, you may have to use it. It is important to be familiar with how to use naloxone.

Facts About Naloxone

Here are some facts about naloxone:

How to get it	Naloxone is available by prescription and through substance abuse treatment programs.
How to use it	Naloxone comes in several forms. Common forms are an intranasal spray or autoinjector (similar to an epinephrine pen). Give naloxone by spraying it into the nose or by injecting it into a muscle with an autoinjector.
Who can give it	Naloxone should only be given by someone who has been trained and can identify an opioid overdose.
When to give it	Naloxone is used to reverse the effects of an opioid overdose. It won't work for other types of drug overdoses.

Actions to Help an Adult With Opioid-Associated Emergency

If you suspect that someone has had an opioid overdose and the person is still responsive, phone 9-1-1 and stay with the person until someone with more advanced training arrives.

If the person becomes unresponsive, follow these steps:

Actions to Help an Adult With Opioid-Associated Emergency
☐ Shout for help.
☐ If someone is nearby, have that person phone 9-1-1 and get the naloxone kit and AED. Use the naloxone as soon as it arrives.
☐ Check for breathing.
☐ If no one is nearby and the person isn't breathing normally or is only gasping, provide CPR. After 5 cycles of CPR, phone 9-1-1 and get the naloxone and AED.
☐ Return to the person and give the naloxone. Check for responsiveness and breathing. • If the person becomes responsive, stop CPR and wait for advanced help to arrive.
☐ If the person continues to be unresponsive, continue CPR and use the AED as soon as it is available.
☐ Continue CPR and using the AED until • Someone else arrives who can take turns providing CPR with you • The person begins to move, speak, blink, or otherwise react • Someone with more advanced training arrives

CPR and AED Use for Children

What You Will Learn

In this section, you will learn when CPR is needed, how to give CPR to a child, and how to use an AED.

Definition of a Child

For the purposes of this course, a child is from 1 year of age to puberty. Signs of puberty include chest or underarm hair in males and any breast development in females. If you are in doubt about whether someone is an adult or child, provide emergency care as if the person is an adult.

The definition of *child* is different when using an AED compared with providing CPR. See "Use an AED" later in this section.

Pediatric Chain of Survival

The AHA pediatric Chain of Survival (Figure 44) shows the most important actions needed to treat cardiac arrests in children that occur outside of a hospital.

During this course, you will learn about the first 3 links of the chain. The fourth and fifth links are advanced care provided by emergency responders and hospital providers who will take over care.

First link 	Preventing injury and sudden cardiac arrest is an important first step in saving children's lives.
Second link 	The sooner that high-quality CPR is started for someone in cardiac arrest, the better the chances of survival.
Third link 	Phoning 9-1-1 as soon as possible so that the child can have emergency care quickly improves outcome.

Remember that seconds count when a child has a cardiac arrest. Wherever you are, take action. The pediatric Chain of Survival starts with you!

Figure 44. The AHA pediatric Chain of Survival for cardiac arrests outside of a hospital.

Respiratory Problems Often Cause Cardiac Arrest in Children

Children usually have healthy hearts. Breathing trouble is often the cause of a child needing CPR. Some other causes are drowning, trauma, and electrical injury. In the pediatric Chain of Survival, preventing cardiac arrest is one of the most important things you can do. This includes prevention of drowning, choking, and other respiratory problems.

Since respiratory problems are often the cause of cardiac arrest in children, if you are alone and do not have a phone nearby, provide CPR for 2 minutes before leaving to phone 9-1-1.

Topics Covered

- Assess and Phone 9-1-1
- Perform High-Quality CPR
- Use an AED
- Putting It All Together: Child High-Quality CPR AED Summary

When you encounter a child who may have had a cardiac arrest, take the following steps to assess the emergency and get help:

- Make sure the scene is safe.
- Tap and shout (check for responsiveness).
- Shout for help.
- Check for breathing.
- Begin CPR, phone 9-1-1, and get an AED.

Depending on the particular circumstance and the resources you have available, you may be able to perform some of these actions at the same time. You might, for example, phone 9-1-1 with your cell phone on speaker mode while checking for breathing.

Make Sure the Scene Is Safe

Before you assess the child, make sure the scene is safe. Look for anything nearby that might hurt you. You can't help if you get hurt too.

As you give care, be aware if anything changes and makes it unsafe for you or the child.

Tap and Shout (Check for Responsiveness)

Tap and shout to check if the child is responsive or unresponsive (Figure 45).

Lean over the child or kneel at his side. Tap his shoulders and ask if he is OK.

If	Then
The child moves, speaks, blinks, or otherwise reacts when you tap him.	• He is *responsive*. • Ask the child if he needs help.
The child doesn't move, speak, blink, or otherwise react when you tap him.	• He is *unresponsive*. • Shout for help so that if others are nearby, they can help you.

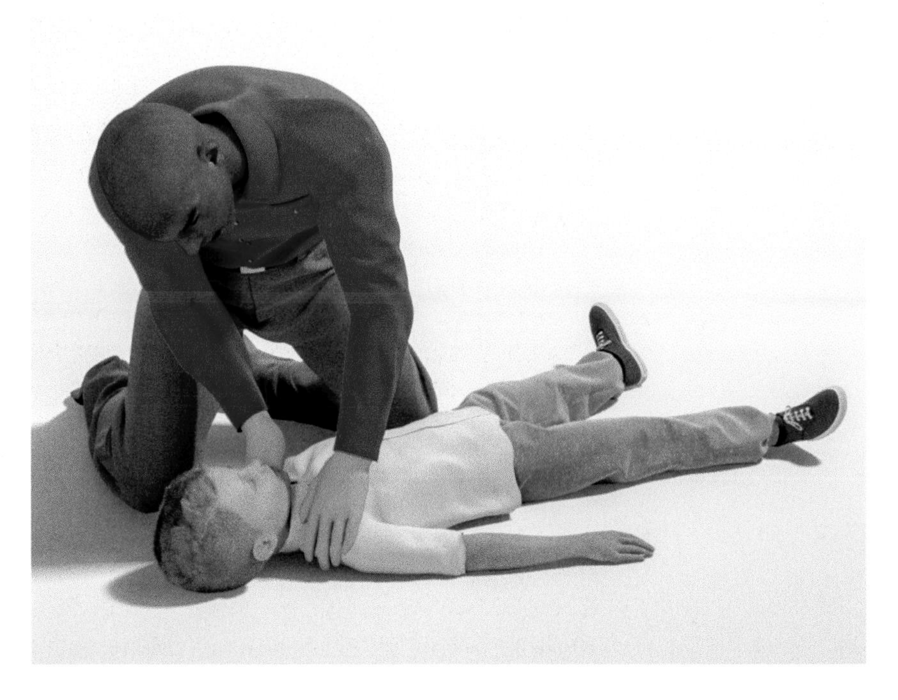

Figure 45. Tap and shout (check for responsiveness).

Shout for Help

In an emergency, the sooner you realize that there's a problem and get additional help, the better it is for the child with a cardiac arrest. When more people are helping, you are able to provide better care to the child.

If the child is unresponsive, shout for help (Figure 46). If someone comes, send that person to phone 9-1-1 and get an AED. If you have a cell phone, phone 9-1-1 and put it on speaker mode.

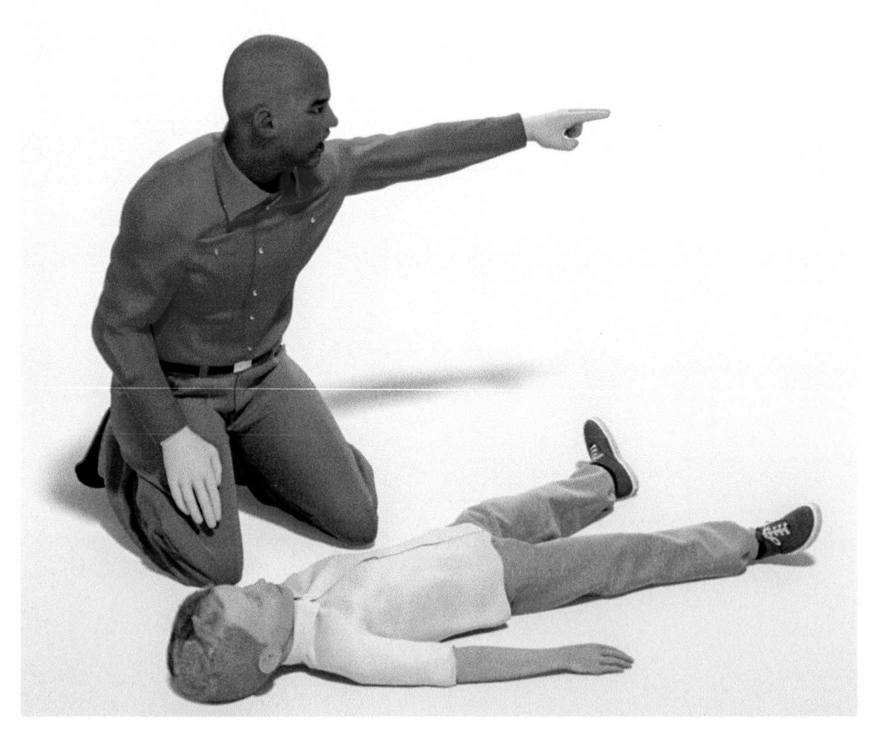

Figure 46. Shout for help.

Check for Breathing

If the child is unresponsive, check for breathing (Figure 47).

Scan the chest from head to chest repeatedly for at least 5 seconds (but no more than 10 seconds) looking for chest rise and fall. If the child is not breathing or is only gasping, he needs CPR. (See "Heartsaver First Aid CPR AED Terms and Concepts" for more information on gasping.)

If	Then
The child is unresponsive and is breathing.	• This child does not need CPR. • Roll him onto his side (if you don't think he has a neck or back injury). This will help keep the airway clear in the event the child vomits. • Stay with the child until advanced help arrives.
The child is unresponsive and not breathing or is only gasping.	• This child needs CPR. • Make sure the child is lying on his back on a firm, flat surface. • Have someone phone 9-1-1, or use your cell phone (or nearby phone), put it on speaker mode, and phone 9-1-1. • Begin CPR. Give 5 sets of 30 compressions and 2 breaths. • After 5 sets of compressions and breaths, phone 9-1-1 and get an AED (if no one has done this yet). As soon as you have an AED, use it.

Remember

Unresponsive
+
No breathing or only gasping
= Provide CPR

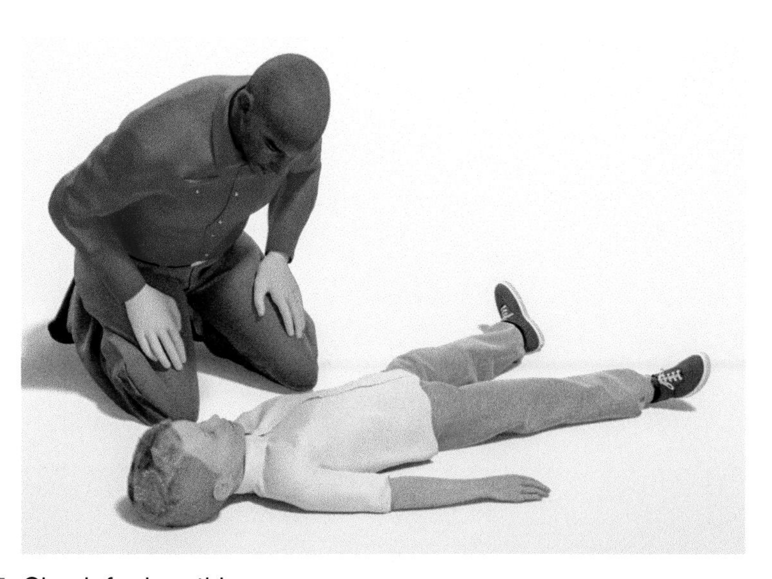

Figure 47. Check for breathing.

Begin CPR, Phone 9-1-1, and Get an AED

If someone comes to help and a cell phone is available

- Ask the person to phone 9-1-1 on the cell phone, put it on speaker mode, and go get an AED while you begin CPR.

If someone comes to help and a cell phone is not available

- Ask the person to go phone 9-1-1 and get an AED while you begin CPR.

If you are alone and have a cell phone or nearby phone

- Phone 9-1-1 and put the phone on speaker mode while you begin CPR.
- Give 5 sets of 30 compressions and 2 breaths.
- Go get an AED.
- Return to the child and continue CPR.

If you are alone and don't have a cell phone

- Give 5 sets of 30 compressions and 2 breaths.
- Go phone 9-1-1 and get an AED.
- Return to the child and continue CPR.

Follow Dispatcher's Instructions

Stay on the phone until the 9-1-1 dispatcher tells you to hang up. Answering the dispatcher's questions will not delay the arrival of help.

The dispatcher will ask you about the emergency—where you are and what has happened. Dispatchers can provide instructions that will help you, such as telling you how to provide CPR, use an AED, or give first aid.

That's why it's important to put the phone on speaker mode after phoning 9-1-1 so that the dispatcher and the person providing CPR can speak to each other.

What to Do If You Are Not Sure

If you think a child needs CPR but you aren't sure, provide CPR because you may save a life. CPR is not likely to cause harm if the child is not in cardiac arrest.

It's better to give CPR to a child who doesn't need it than not to give it to a child who does need it.

Summary

Here is a summary of how to assess the emergency and get help when you encounter an ill or injured child:

Assess and Get Help
☐ Make sure the scene is safe.
☐ Tap and shout (check for responsiveness). • If the child is *responsive,* ask him if he needs help. • If the child is *unresponsive,* go to the next step.
☐ Shout for help.
☐ Check for breathing. • If the child is breathing, stay with the child until advanced help arrives. • If the child is *not* breathing or only gasping, begin CPR and use an AED. See the next steps.

Begin CPR, Phone 9-1-1, and Get an AED
☐ Make sure the child is lying on his back on a firm, flat surface.
☐ Quickly move clothes out of the way.
☐ Begin CPR, phone 9-1-1, and get an AED. *If someone comes to help and a cell phone is available* • Ask the person to phone 9-1-1 on the cell phone, put it on speaker mode, and go get an AED while you begin CPR. *If someone comes to help and a cell phone is not available* • Ask the person to go phone 9-1-1 and get an AED while you begin CPR. *If you are alone and have a cell phone or nearby phone* • Phone 9-1-1 and put the phone on speaker mode while you begin CPR. • Give 5 sets of 30 compressions and 2 breaths. • Go get an AED. • Return to the child and continue CPR. *If you are alone and don't have a cell phone* • Give 5 sets of 30 compressions and 2 breaths. • Go phone 9-1-1 and get an AED. • Return to the child and continue CPR.
☐ Continue providing CPR and using the AED until • Someone else arrives who can take turns providing CPR with you • The child begins to move, speak, blink, or otherwise react • Someone with more advanced training arrives

Learning how to perform high-quality CPR is important. The better the CPR skills are performed, the better the chances of survival.

CPR Skills

CPR has 2 main skills:

- Providing compressions
- Giving breaths

You will learn how to perform these skills for a child in cardiac arrest in this section.

Provide Compressions

A compression is the act of pushing hard and fast on the chest. When a child's heart stops, blood stops flowing through the body. When you push on the chest, you pump blood to the brain and heart.

To perform high-quality compressions, make sure that you

- Provide compressions that are deep enough
- Provide compressions that are fast enough
- Let the chest come back up to its normal position after each compression
- Try not to interrupt compressions for more than 10 seconds, even when you give breaths

Compression depth is an important part of providing high-quality compressions. You need to push hard enough to pump blood through the body. It's better to push too hard than not hard enough. People are often afraid of causing a child injury by providing compressions, but injury is unlikely.

Compression Technique

When providing compressions for a child, use 1 hand (Figure 48). If you can't push down at least one third the depth of the child's chest (or about 2 inches) with 1 hand, use 2 hands to compress the chest (Figure 49).

Here is how to provide compressions for a child during CPR:

How to Provide Compressions for a Child During CPR
☐ Make sure the child is lying on his back on a firm, flat surface.
☐ Quickly move clothes out of the way.
☐ Use either 1 hand or 2 hands to give compressions. • **1 hand:** Put the heel of one hand on the center of the chest (over the lower half of the breastbone). • **2 hands:** Put the heel of one hand on the center of the chest (over the lower half of the breastbone). Put your other hand on top of the first hand.
☐ Push straight down at least one third the depth of the chest or about 2 inches.
☐ Push at a rate of 100 to 120 compressions per minute. Count the compressions out loud.
☐ Let the chest come back up to its normal position after each compression.

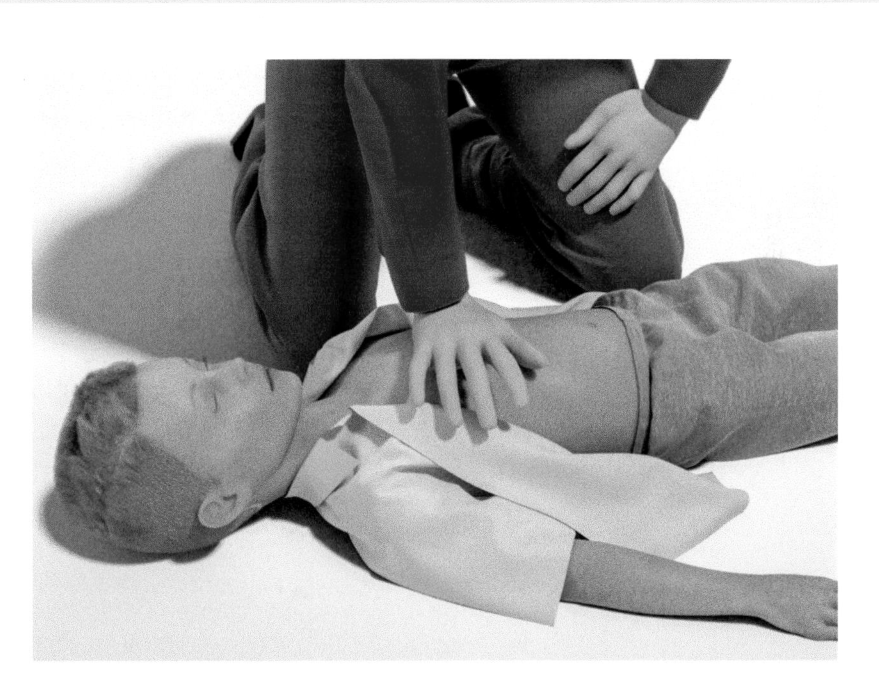

Figure 48. Using 1 hand to give compressions to a child.

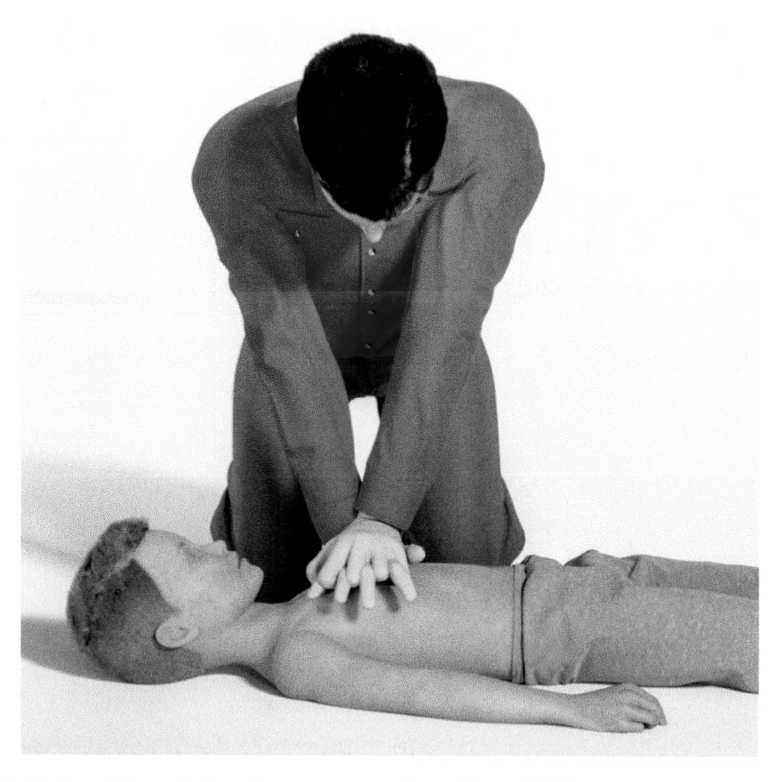

Figure 49. Using 2 hands to give compressions to a child.

Switch Rescuers to Avoid Fatigue

Performing chest compressions correctly is hard work. The more tired you become, the less effective your compressions will be.

If someone else knows CPR, you can take turns providing CPR (Figure 50). Switch rescuers about every 2 minutes, or sooner if you get tired, moving quickly to keep any pauses in compressions as short as possible.

Remind other rescuers to perform high-quality CPR as described in the box labeled "How to Provide Compressions for a Child During CPR."

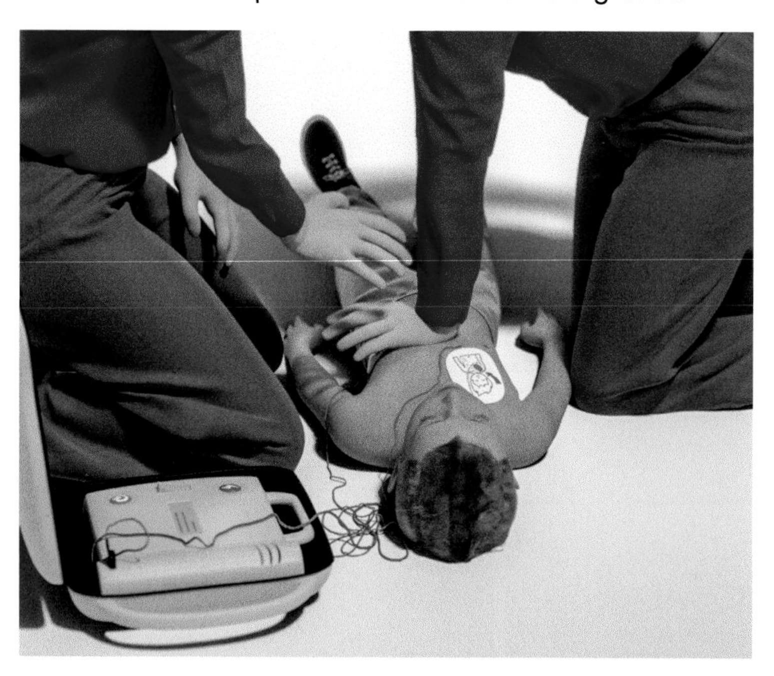

Figure 50. Switch rescuers about every 2 minutes to avoid fatigue.

Give Breaths

The second skill of CPR is giving breaths. After each set of 30 compressions, you will need to give 2 breaths. Breaths may be given with or without a barrier device, such as a pocket mask or face shield.

When you give breaths, the breaths need to make the chest rise visibly. When you can see the chest rise, you know you have delivered an effective breath.

Open the Airway

Before giving breaths, open the airway (Figure 51). This lifts the tongue from the back of the throat to make sure your breaths get air into the lungs.

Follow these steps to open the airway:

How to Open the Airway
☐ Put one hand on the forehead and the fingers of your other hand on the bony part of the chin (Figure 51).
☐ Tilt the head back and lift the chin.

Avoid pressing into the soft part of the neck or under the chin because this might block the airway.

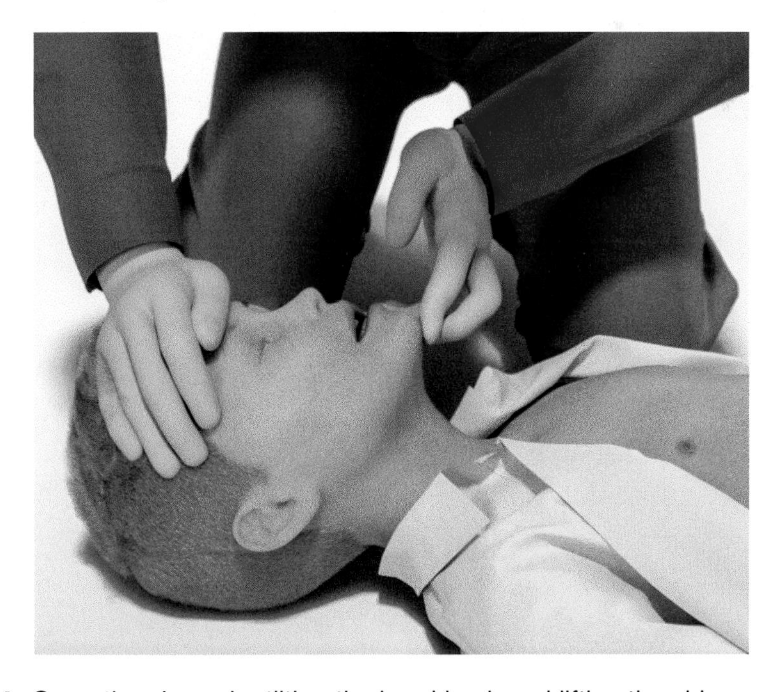

Figure 51. Open the airway by tilting the head back and lifting the chin.

Give Breaths Without a Pocket Mask

If you choose to give someone breaths without a barrier device, it is usually quite safe because there is very little chance that you will catch a disease.

As you give each breath, look at the child's chest to see if it begins to rise. For small children, you will not need to blow as much as for larger children. Actually seeing the chest begin to rise is the best way to know that your breaths are effective.

Follow these steps to give breaths without a pocket mask or face shield (Figure 52):

How to Give Breaths (Without a Mask)
☐ While holding the airway open, pinch the nose closed with your thumb and forefinger.
☐ Take a normal breath. Cover the child's mouth with your mouth.
☐ Give 2 breaths (blow for 1 second for each). Watch for the chest to begin to rise as you give each breath.
☐ Try not to interrupt compressions for more than 10 seconds.

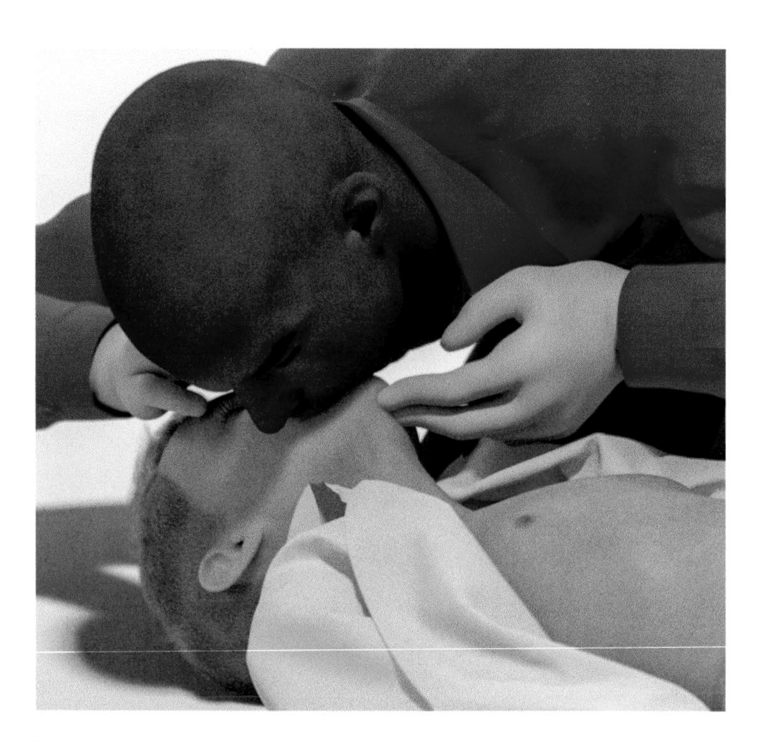

Figure 52. Cover the child's mouth with your mouth.

What to Do If the Chest Doesn't Rise

It takes a little practice to give breaths correctly. If you give someone a breath and the chest doesn't rise, do the following:

- Allow the head to go back to its normal position.
- Open the airway again by tilting the head back and lifting the chin.
- Then, give another breath. Make sure the chest rises.

Minimize Interruptions in Chest Compressions

If you have been unable to give 2 effective breaths in 10 seconds, go back to pushing hard and fast on the chest. Try to give breaths again after every 30 compressions.

Don't interrupt compressions for more than 10 seconds.

Use a Pocket Mask

You may give breaths with or without a barrier device, such as a pocket mask. Barrier devices are made of plastic and fit over the person's mouth and nose (Figure 53). They protect the rescuer from blood, vomit, or disease. Your instructor may discuss other types of barrier devices, like face shields, which can be used when giving breaths.

If you're in the workplace, your employer may provide personal protective equipment, including pocket masks or face shields, for use during CPR.

There are many different kinds of pocket masks as well as different sizes for adults, children, and infants. So, make sure you're using the right size. You may need to put a pocket mask together before you use it.

Give Breaths With a Pocket Mask

Follow these steps to give breaths with a pocket mask (Figure 53):

How to Give Breaths With a Pocket Mask
☐ Put the mask over the child's mouth and nose. • If the mask has a pointed end, put the narrow end of the mask on the bridge of the nose; position the wide end so that it covers the mouth.
☐ Tilt the head and lift the chin while pressing the mask against the child's face. It is important to make an airtight seal between the child's face and the mask while you lift the chin to keep the airway open.
☐ Give 2 breaths (blow for 1 second for each). Watch for the chest to begin to rise as you give each breath.
☐ Try not to interrupt compressions for more than 10 seconds.

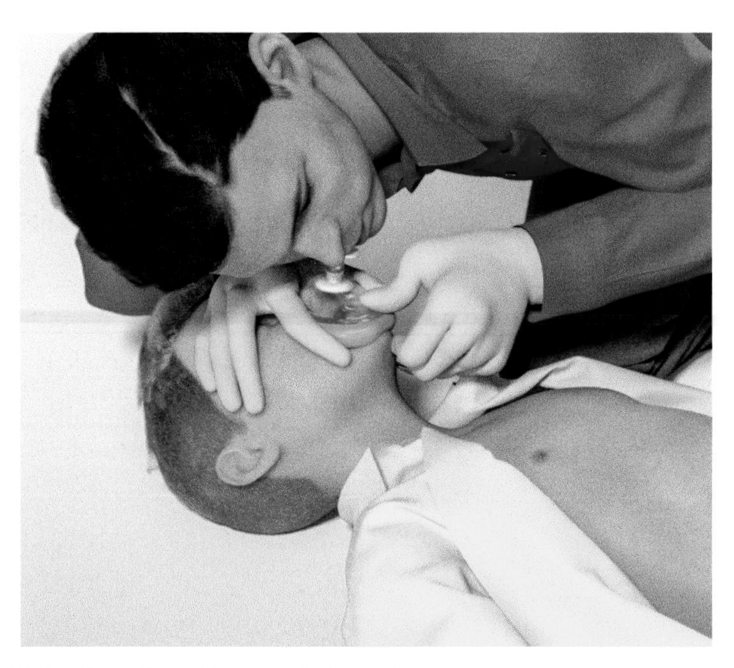

Figure 53. Giving breaths with a pocket mask.

Give Sets of 30 Compressions and 2 Breaths

When providing CPR, give sets of 30 compressions and 2 breaths.

How to Give Sets of Compressions and Breaths to a Child
☐ Make sure the child is lying on his back on a firm, flat surface.
☐ Quickly move clothes out of the way.
☐ Give 30 chest compressions. • Use either 1 hand or 2 hands to give compressions. • **1 hand:** Put the heel of one hand on the center of the chest (over the lower half of the breastbone). • **2 hands:** Put the heel of one hand on the center of the chest (over the lower half of the breastbone). Put your other hand on top of the first hand. • Push straight down at least one third the depth of the chest or about 2 inches. • Push at a rate of 100 to 120 compressions per minute. Count the compressions out loud. • Let the chest come back up to its normal position after each compression.
☐ After 30 compressions, give 2 breaths. • Open the airway and give 2 breaths (blow for 1 second for each). Watch for the chest to begin to rise as you give each breath. • Try not to interrupt compressions for more than 10 seconds.

CPR combined with using an AED provides the best chance of saving a life. If possible, use an AED every time you provide CPR.

AEDs can be used for children and infants, as well as adults.

- Some AEDs can deliver a smaller shock dose for children and infants if you use child pads or a child-cable key or switch.
- If the AED can deliver the smaller shock dose, use it for infants and children less than 8 years of age.
- If the AED cannot deliver a child shock dose, you can use the adult pads and give an adult shock dose for infants and children less than 8 years of age.

AEDs are safe, accurate, and easy to use. Once you turn on the AED, follow the prompts. The AED will analyze if the child needs a shock and will automatically give one or tell you when to give one.

Turn on the AED

To use an AED, turn it on by either pushing the "on" button or lifting the lid (Figure 54). Once you turn on the AED, you will hear prompts, which will tell you everything you need to do.

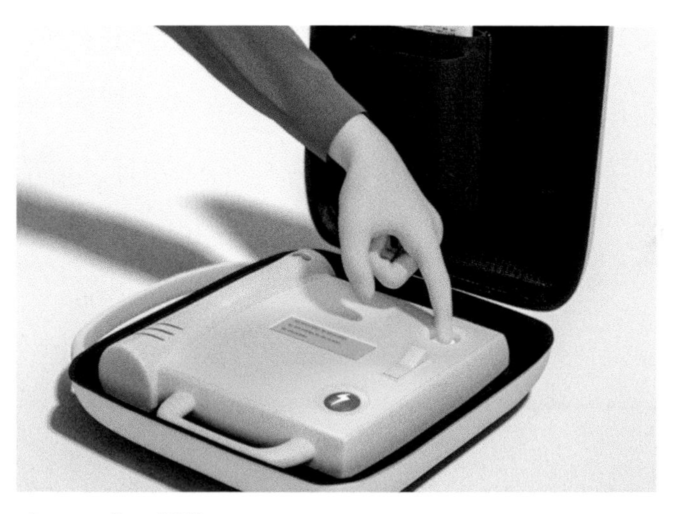

Figure 54. Turning on the AED.

Attach the Pads

Many AEDs have pads for adults and a child pad-cable system or key for children and infants.

- Use child pads if the child or infant is less than 8 years old. If child pads are not available, use adult pads.
- Use adult pads if the child is 8 years old or older.

Before you place the pads, quickly scan the child to see if there are any special situations that might require additional steps. See "Special Situations" below.

Peel away the backing from the pads. Follow the pad placement as shown on the images on the pads or package. Attach the pads to the child's bare chest (Figure 55).

When you put the pads on the chest, make sure they don't touch each other. If the child's chest is small, the pads may overlap. In this case you may need to put one pad on the child's chest and the other on the child's back.

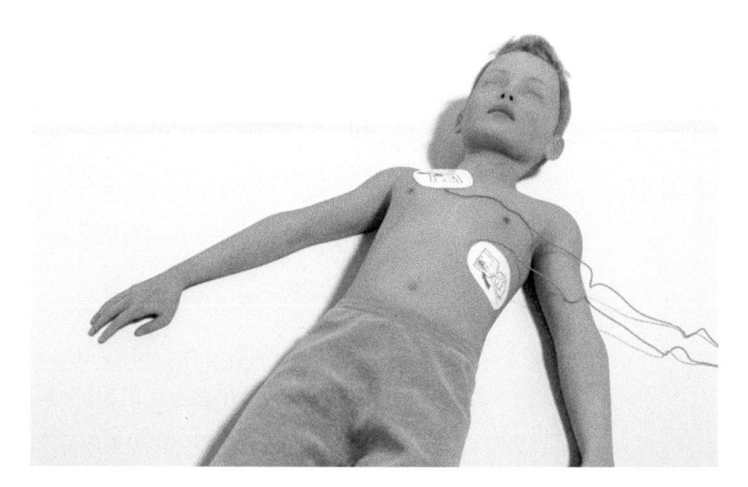

Figure 55. Place pads on a child by following the pictures on the pads.

Clear the Child if a Shock Is Advised

Let the AED analyze the heart rhythm. If the AED advises a shock, it will tell you to stay clear of the child. If so, then loudly state, "Clear." Make sure that no one is touching the child just before you push the "shock" button (Figure 56).

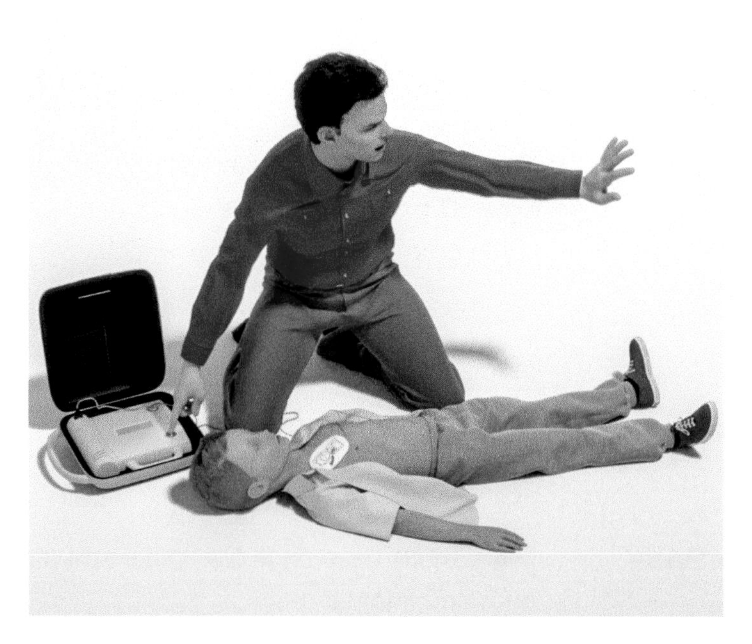

Figure 56. Make sure that no one is touching the child just before you push the "shock" button.

Steps for Using the AED for a Child

Use the AED as soon as it is available. Here are the steps for using the AED for a child:

How to Use an AED for a Child
☐ Turn the AED on and follow the prompts. • Turn it on by pushing the "on" button or lifting the lid (Figure 54). • Follow the prompts, which will tell you everything you need to do.
☐ Attach the pads. • Use child pads if the child is less than 8 years old. If child pads are not available, use adult pads. • Use adult pads if the child is 8 years old or older. • Peel away the backing from the pads. • Following the pictures on the pads, attach them to the child's bare chest (Figure 55). Make sure the pads don't touch each other.
☐ Let the AED analyze. • Loudly state, "Clear," and make sure that no one is touching the child. • The AED will analyze the heart rhythm. • If a shock is not needed, resume CPR.
☐ Deliver a shock if needed (Figure 56). • Loudly state, "Clear," and make sure that no one is touching the child. • Push the "shock" button. • Immediately resume CPR.

Special Situations

There are some special situations that you may need to consider before placing AED pads. Although it is not very common, you may encounter a medicine patch or a device on a child, which may interfere with the AED pad placement.

Quickly scan the child to see if he has any of the following *before* applying the pads:

If the victim…	Then
Is lying in water	• Quickly move the victim to a dry area.
Is lying on snow or in a small puddle	• You may use the AED (the chest doesn't have to be completely dry). • If the chest is covered with water or sweat, quickly wipe it before attaching the pads.
Has water on the chest	• Quickly wipe the chest dry before attaching the pads.
Has an implanted defibrillator or pacemaker	• Don't put the AED pad directly over the implanted device. • Follow the normal steps for operating an AED.

(continued)

(continued)

Has a medicine patch where you need to place an AED pad	• Don't put the AED pad directly over a medicine patch. • Use protective gloves. • Remove the medicated patch. • Wipe the area clean. • Attach the AED pads.

Continue Providing CPR and Using the AED

As soon as the AED gives the shock, immediately resume chest compressions. Continue to follow the AED prompts, which will guide the rescue.

Provide CPR and use the AED until

- Someone else arrives who can take turns providing CPR with you
- The child begins to move, speak, blink, or otherwise react
- Someone with more advanced training arrives

Putting It All Together: Child High-Quality CPR AED Summary

Children usually have healthy hearts. Often, a child's heart stops because the child can't breathe or is having trouble breathing. As a result, it's very important to give breaths as well as compressions to a child.

Compressions are still very important to deliver blood flow and are the core of CPR. Try not to interrupt chest compressions for more than 10 seconds when you give breaths.

Assess and Get Help
☐ Make sure the scene is safe.
☐ Tap and shout (check for responsiveness). • If the child is *responsive,* ask him if he needs help. • If the child is *unresponsive,* go to the next step.
☐ Shout for help.
☐ Check for breathing. • If the child is breathing, stay with the child until advanced help arrives. • If the child is *not* breathing or only gasping, begin CPR and use the AED. See the next steps.

Begin CPR, Phone 9-1-1, and Get an AED

☐ Begin CPR, phone 9-1-1, and get an AED.

If someone comes to help and a cell phone is available

- Ask the person to phone 9-1-1 on the cell phone, put it on speaker mode, and go get an AED while you begin CPR.

If someone comes to help and a cell phone is not available

- Ask the person to go phone 9-1-1 and get an AED while you begin CPR.

If you are alone and have a cell phone or nearby phone

- Phone 9-1-1 and put the phone on speaker mode while you begin CPR.
- Give 5 sets of 30 compressions and 2 breaths.
- Go get an AED.
- Return to the child and continue CPR.

If you are alone and don't have a cell phone

- Give 5 sets of 30 compressions and 2 breaths.
- Then, go phone 9-1-1 and get an AED.
- Return to the child and continue CPR.

Provide High-Quality CPR

When providing CPR, you give sets of 30 compressions and 2 breaths.

☐ Make sure the child is lying on his back on a firm, flat surface.

☐ Quickly move clothes out of the way.

☐ Give 30 chest compressions.

- Use either 1 hand or 2 hands to give compressions.
  - **1 hand:** Put the heel of one hand on the center of the chest (over the lower half of the breastbone).
  - **2 hands:** Put the heel of one hand on the center of the chest (over the lower half of the breastbone). Put your other hand on top of the first hand.
- Push straight down at least one third the depth of the chest or about 2 inches.
- Push at a rate of 100 to 120 compressions per minute. Count the compressions out loud.
- Let the chest come back up to its normal position after each compression.

☐ After 30 compressions, give 2 breaths.

- Open the airway and give 2 breaths (blow for 1 second for each). Watch for the chest to begin to rise as you give each breath.
- Try not to interrupt compressions for more than 10 seconds.

(continued)

(continued)

- ☐ Use an AED as soon as it is available.
  - Turn the AED on and follow the prompts.
  - Attach the pads.
    - Use child pads if the child is less than 8 years old. If child pads are not available, use adult pads.
    - Use adult pads if the child is 8 years old or older.
  - Let the AED analyze.
  - Make sure no one is touching the child, and deliver a shock if advised.

- ☐ Provide CPR and use the AED until
  - Someone else arrives who can take turns providing CPR with you
  - The child begins to move, speak, blink, or otherwise react
  - Someone with more advanced training arrives and takes over

CPR for Infants

What You Will Learn

In this section, you will learn when CPR is needed, how to give CPR to an infant, and how to use an AED.

Definition of an Infant

For the purposes of this course, an infant is less than 1 year old.

Differences in CPR Between an Infant and a Child

Because infants are so small, there are some differences between infants, children, and adults in how CPR is performed. When providing compressions on an infant, you use only 2 fingers of 1 hand—versus 1 or 2 hands for a child and 2 hands for an adult.

Also, for an infant, you should push down about 1½ inches at the rate of 100 to 120 compressions per minute.

Topics Covered

- Assess and Phone 9-1-1
- Perform High-Quality CPR
- Use an AED
- Putting It All Together: Infant High-Quality CPR Summary

When you encounter an infant who may have had a cardiac arrest, take the following steps to assess the emergency and get help:

- Make sure the scene is safe.
- Tap and shout (check for responsiveness).
- Shout for help.
- Check for breathing.
- Begin CPR, phone 9-1-1, and get an AED.

Depending on the particular circumstance and the resources you have available, you may be able to perform some of these actions at the same time. You might, for example, phone 9-1-1 with your cell phone on speaker mode while checking for breathing.

Make Sure the Scene Is Safe

Before you assess the infant, make sure the scene is safe. Look for anything nearby that might hurt you. You can't help if you get hurt too.

As you give care, be aware if anything changes and makes it unsafe for you or the infant.

Tap and Shout (Check for Responsiveness)

Tap and shout to check if the infant is responsive or unresponsive (Figure 57).

Tap the infant's foot and shout his name.

If	Then
The infant moves, cries, blinks, or otherwise reacts when you tap him.	• He is *responsive;* continue first aid care.
The infant doesn't move, cry, blink, or otherwise react when you tap him.	• He is *unresponsive*. • Shout for help so that if others are nearby, they can help you.

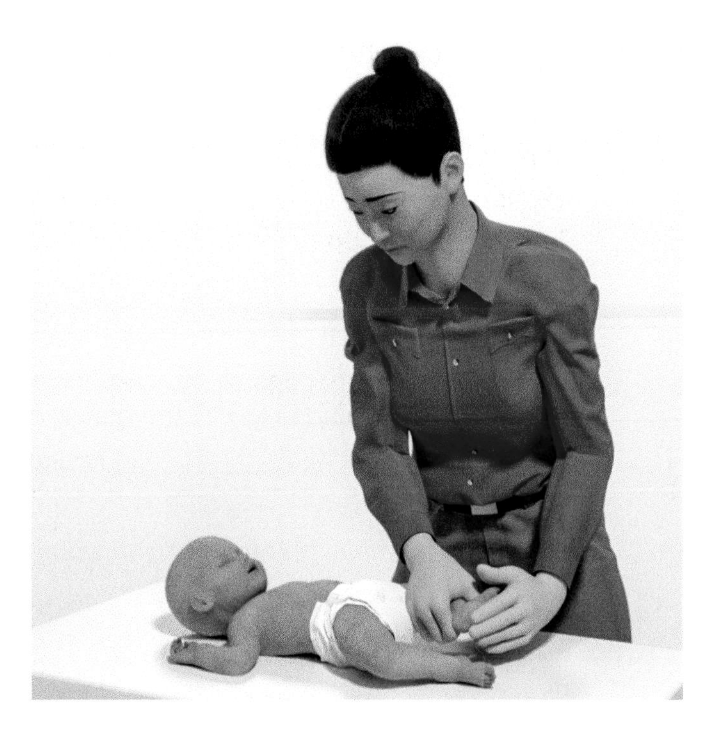

Figure 57. Tap and shout (check for responsiveness).

Shout for Help

In an emergency, the sooner you realize that there's a problem and get additional help, the better it is for the infant with a cardiac arrest. When more people are helping, you are able to provide better care to the infant.

If the infant is unresponsive, shout for help (Figure 58). If someone comes, send that person to phone 9-1-1 and get an AED. If you have a cell phone, phone 9-1-1 and put it on speaker mode.

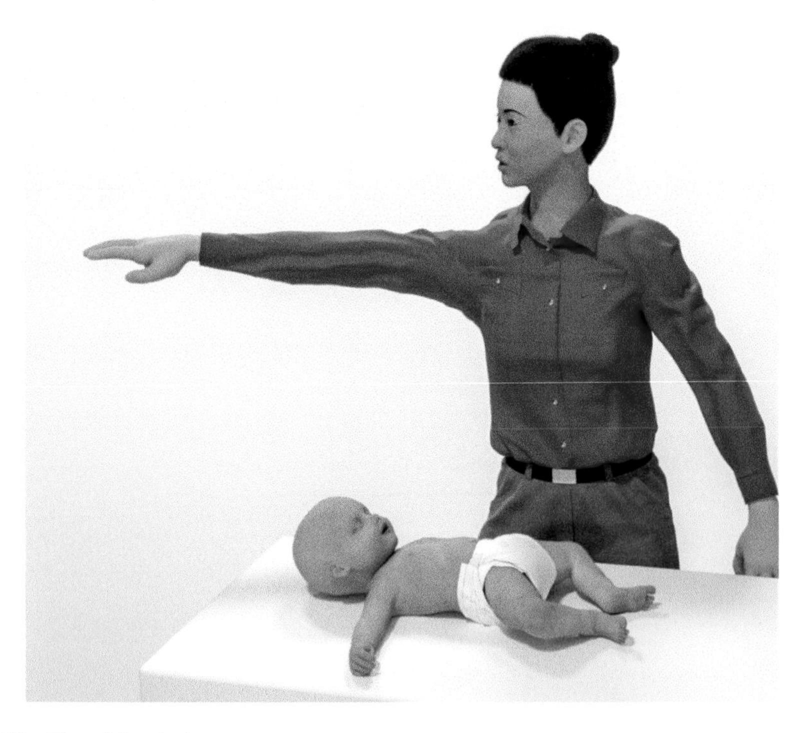

Figure 58. Shout for help.

Check for Breathing

If the infant is unresponsive, check for breathing (Figure 59).

Scan the chest from head to chest repeatedly for at least 5 seconds (but no more than 10 seconds) looking for chest rise and fall. If the infant is not breathing or is only gasping, he needs CPR. (See "Heartsaver First Aid CPR AED Terms and Concepts" for more information on gasping.)

If	Then
The infant is unresponsive and is breathing.	• This infant does not need CPR. • Roll him onto his side (if you don't think he has a neck or back injury). This will help keep the airway clear in the event the infant vomits. • Stay with the infant until advanced help arrives.
The infant is unresponsive and not breathing or is only gasping.	• This infant needs CPR. • Make sure the infant is lying on his back on a firm, flat surface. • Have someone phone 9-1-1, or use your cell phone (or nearby phone), put it on speaker mode, and phone 9-1-1. • Begin CPR. Give 5 sets of 30 compressions and 2 breaths. • After 5 sets of compressions and breaths, phone 9-1-1 and get an AED (if no one has done this yet). As soon as you have an AED, use it.

Remember

Unresponsive + No breathing or only gasping = Provide CPR

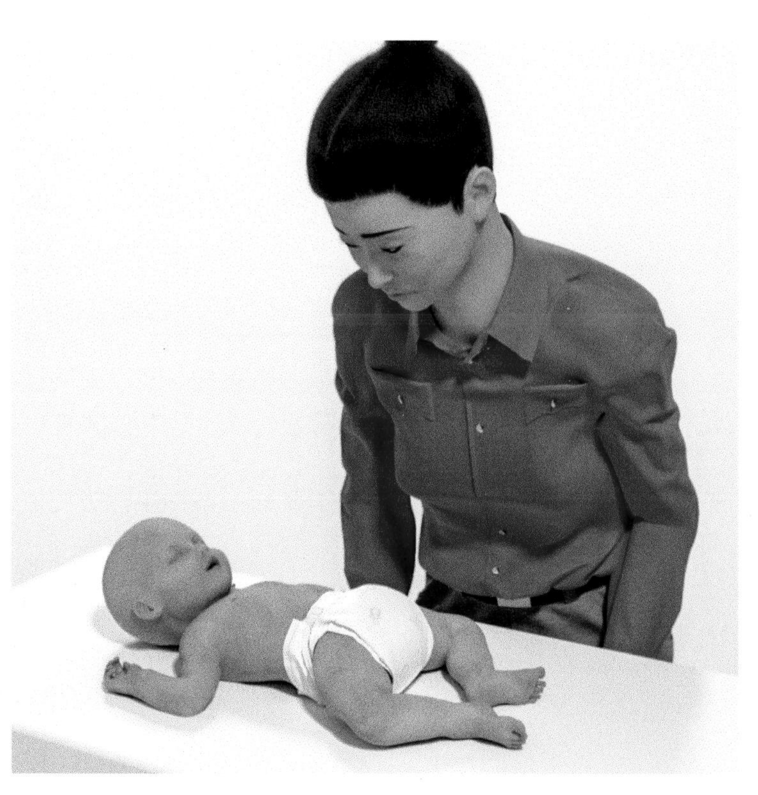

Figure 59. Check for breathing.

Begin CPR, Phone 9-1-1, and Get an AED

If someone comes to help and a cell phone is available

- Ask the person to phone 9-1-1 on the cell phone, put it on speaker mode, and go get an AED while you begin CPR.

If someone comes to help and a cell phone is not available

- Ask the person to go phone 9-1-1 and get an AED while you begin CPR.

If you are alone and have a cell phone or nearby phone

- Phone 9-1-1 and put the phone on speaker mode while you begin CPR.
- Give 5 sets of 30 compressions and 2 breaths.
- Go get an AED.*
- Return to the infant and continue CPR.

If you are alone and don't have a cell phone

- Give 5 sets of 30 compressions and 2 breaths.
- Go phone 9-1-1 and get an AED.*
- Return to the infant and continue CPR.

*If the infant isn't injured and you're alone, after 5 sets of 30 compressions and 2 breaths, you may carry the infant with you to phone 9-1-1 and get an AED (Figure 60).

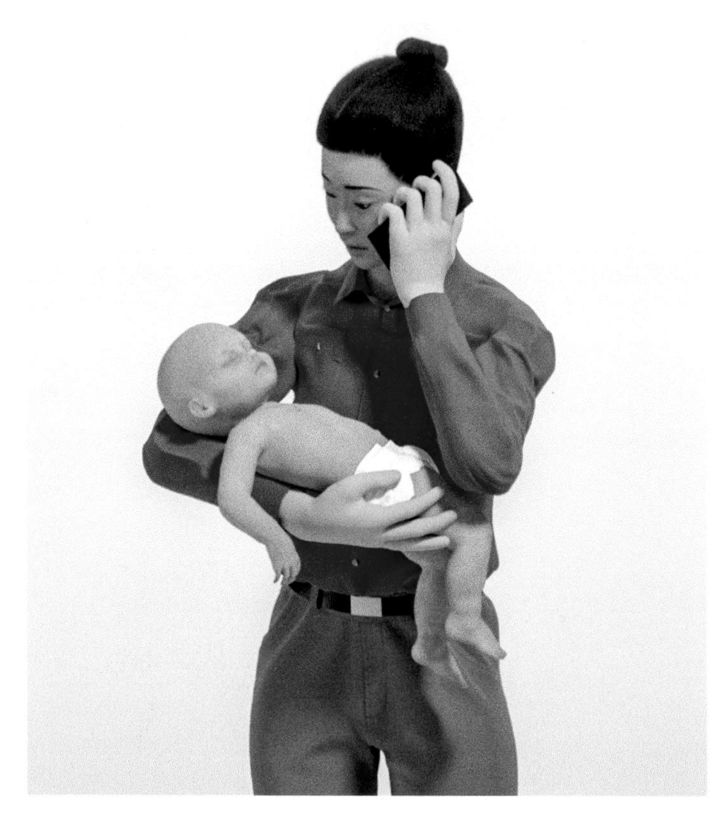

Figure 60. You may carry the infant with you to phone 9-1-1 and get an AED.

Follow Dispatcher's Instructions

Stay on the phone until the 9-1-1 dispatcher tells you to hang up. Answering the dispatcher's questions will not delay the arrival of help.

The dispatcher will ask you about the emergency—where you are and what has happened. Dispatchers can provide instructions that will help you, such as telling you how to provide CPR, use an AED, or give first aid.

That's why it's important to put the phone on speaker mode after phoning 9-1-1 so that the dispatcher and the person providing CPR can speak to each other.

What to Do If You Are Not Sure

If you think an infant needs CPR but you aren't sure, provide CPR because you may save a life. CPR is not likely to cause harm if the infant is not in cardiac arrest.

It's better to give CPR to an infant who doesn't need it than not to give it to an infant who does need it.

Summary

Here is a summary of how to assess the emergency and get help when you encounter an ill or injured infant:

Assess and Get Help
☐ Make sure the scene is safe.
☐ Tap and shout (check for responsiveness). • If the infant is *responsive,* continue first aid care. • If the infant is *unresponsive,* go to the next step.
☐ Shout for help.
☐ Check for breathing. • If the infant is breathing, stay with the infant until advanced help arrives. • If the infant is *not* breathing or only gasping, begin CPR and use an AED. See the next steps.

Begin CPR, Phone 9-1-1, and Get an AED
When providing CPR, you give sets of 30 compressions and 2 breaths.
☐ Make sure the infant is lying on his back on a firm, flat surface.
☐ Quickly move clothes out of the way.
☐ Begin CPR, phone 9-1-1, and get an AED.

If someone comes to help and a cell phone is available

- Ask the person to phone 9-1-1 on the cell phone, put it on speaker mode, and go get an AED while you begin CPR.

If someone comes to help and a cell phone is not available

- Ask the person to go phone 9-1-1 and get an AED while you begin CPR.

If you are alone and have a cell phone or nearby phone

- Phone 9-1-1 and put the phone on speaker mode while you begin CPR.
- Give 5 sets of 30 compressions and 2 breaths.
- Go get an AED.*
- Return to the infant and continue CPR.

If you are alone and don't have a cell phone

- Give 5 sets of 30 compressions and 2 breaths.
- Go phone 9-1-1 and get an AED.*
- Return to the infant and continue CPR.

*If the infant isn't injured and you're alone, after 5 sets of 30 compressions and 2 breaths, you may carry the infant with you to phone 9-1-1 and get an AED.

(continued)

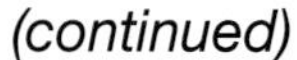

- [ ] Continue providing CPR and using the AED until
  - Someone else arrives who can take turns providing CPR with you
  - The infant begins to move, cry, blink, or otherwise react
  - Someone with more advanced training arrives

Perform High-Quality CPR

Learning how to perform high-quality CPR is important. The better the CPR skills are performed, the better the chances of survival.

CPR Skills

CPR has 2 main skills:

- Providing compressions
- Giving breaths

You will learn how to perform these skills for an infant in cardiac arrest in this section.

Provide Compressions

A compression is the act of pushing hard and fast on the chest. When an infant's heart stops, blood stops flowing through the body. When you push on the chest, you pump blood to the brain and heart.

Pushing hard and fast when providing compressions is just as important with infants as it is with children and adults.

Compressions are the most important part of CPR. To perform high-quality CPR, make sure that you

- Provide compressions that are deep enough
- Provide compressions that are fast enough
- Let the chest come back up to its normal position after each compression
- Try not to interrupt compressions for more than 10 seconds, even when you give breaths

Compression depth is an important part of providing high-quality compressions. You need to push hard enough to pump blood through the body. It's better to push too hard than not hard enough. People are often afraid of causing an infant injury by providing compressions, but injury is unlikely.

Compression Technique

One of the main differences in infant CPR is that you use just 2 fingers in providing compressions. Look at Figure 61 to see the correct placement of your fingers on the baby's chest. Place 2 fingers of 1 hand on the breastbone, just below the nipple line. Push straight down at least one third the depth of the chest or about 1½ inches.

Here is how to provide compressions for an infant during CPR:

How to Provide Compressions for an Infant During CPR
☐ Make sure the infant is lying on his back on a firm, flat surface.
☐ Quickly move clothes out of the way.
☐ Use 2 fingers of 1 hand to give compressions. Place them on the breastbone, just below the nipple line (Figure 61).
☐ Push straight down at least one third the depth of the chest or about 1½ inches.
☐ Push at a rate of 100 to 120 compressions per minute. Count the compressions out loud.
☐ Let the chest come back up to its normal position after each compression.

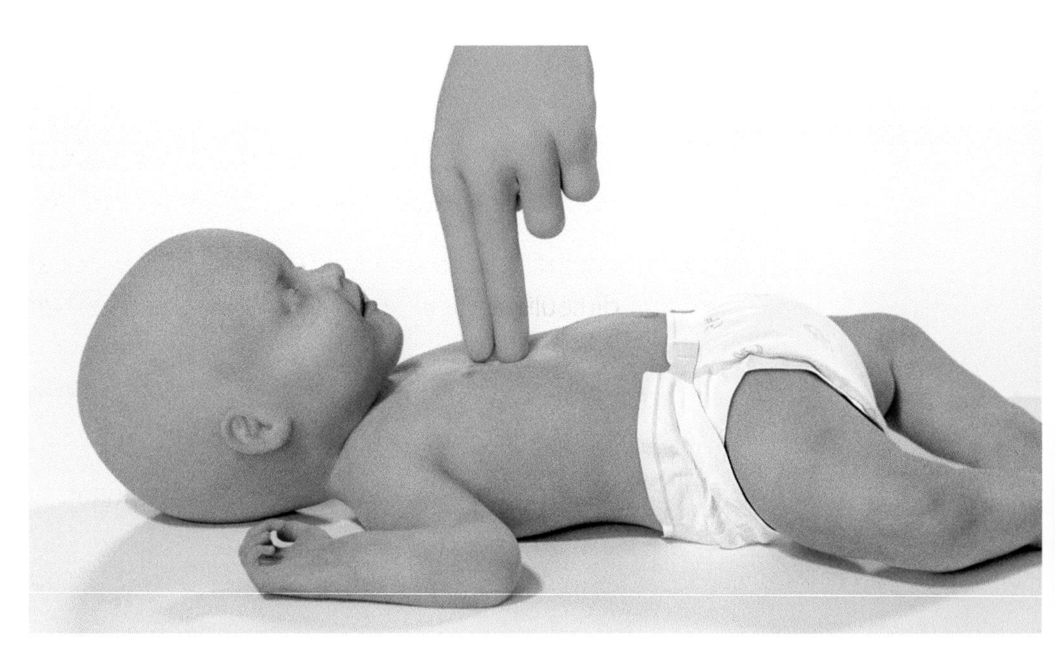

Figure 61. Use 2 fingers of 1 hand to give compressions. Place them on the breastbone, just below the nipple line. Avoid the tip of the breastbone.

Switch Rescuers to Avoid Fatigue

Performing chest compressions correctly is hard work. The more tired you become, the less effective your compressions will be.

If someone else knows CPR, you can take turns providing CPR. Switch rescuers about every 2 minutes, or sooner if you get tired, moving quickly to keep any pauses in compressions as short as possible.

Remind other rescuers to perform high-quality CPR as described in the box labeled "How to Provide Compressions for an Infant During CPR."

Give Breaths

The second skill of CPR is giving breaths. After each set of 30 compressions, you will need to give 2 breaths. Breaths may be given with or without a barrier device, such as a pocket mask or face shield.

Infants often have healthy hearts, but even an infant's heart can stop beating if he can't breathe or has trouble breathing. So, it's very important to give breaths as well as compressions to an infant who needs CPR.

When you give breaths, the breaths need to make the chest rise visibly. When you can see the chest rise, you know you have delivered an effective breath.

Open the Airway

Before giving breaths, open the airway. This lifts the tongue from the back of the throat to make sure your breaths get air into the lungs.

Opening the infant's airway too far can actually *close* the infant's airway, making it difficult to get air inside. Follow these steps to make sure you open the infant's airway correctly:

How to Open the Airway
☐ Put one hand on the forehead and the fingers of your other hand on the bony part of the chin.
☐ Tilt the head back and lift the chin.

Avoid pressing into the soft part of the neck or under the chin because this might block the airway. Also, don't push the head back too far. This might close the airway as well.

Give Breaths Without a Pocket Mask

If you choose to give someone breaths without a barrier device, it is usually quite safe because there is very little chance that you will catch a disease.

As you give each breath, look at the infant's chest to see if it begins to rise. You will not need to blow as much as for a larger child. Actually seeing the chest begin to rise is the best way to know that your breaths are effective.

Follow these steps to give breaths without a pocket mask or face shield (Figure 62):

How to Give Breaths (Without a Pocket Mask)
☐ While holding the airway open, take a normal breath. Cover the infant's mouth and nose with your mouth. If you have difficulty making an effective seal, try either a mouth-to-mouth or a mouth-to-nose breath. • If you use the mouth-to-mouth technique, pinch the nose closed. • If you use the mouth-to-nose technique, close the mouth.
☐ Give 2 breaths (blow for 1 second for each). Watch for the chest to begin to rise as you give each breath.
☐ Try not to interrupt compressions for more than 10 seconds.

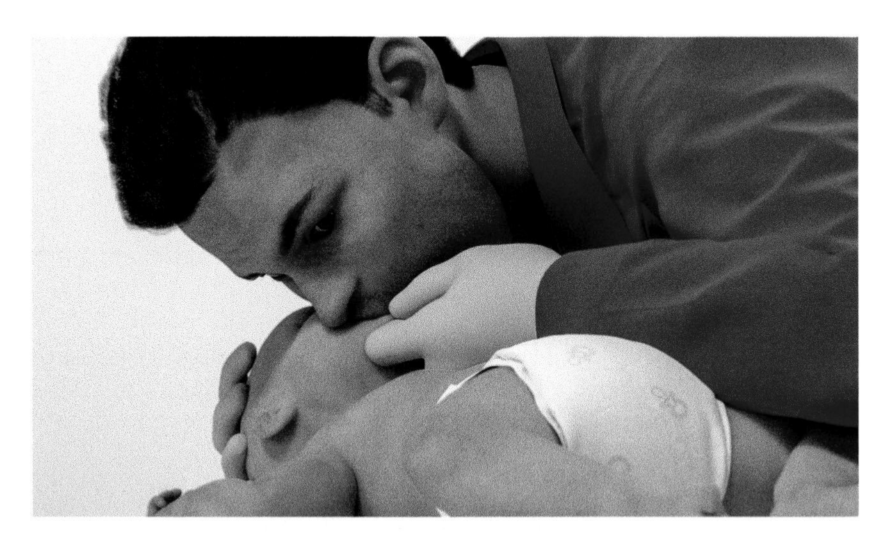

Figure 62. Cover the infant's mouth and nose with your mouth.

What to Do If the Chest Doesn't Rise

It takes a little practice to give breaths correctly. If you give someone a breath and the chest doesn't rise, do the following:

- Allow the head to go back to its normal position.
- Open the airway again by tilting the head back and lifting the chin.
- Then, give another breath. Make sure the chest rises.

Minimize Interruptions in Chest Compressions

If you have been unable to give 2 effective breaths in 10 seconds, go back to pushing hard and fast on the chest. Try to give breaths again after every 30 compressions.

Don't interrupt compressions for more than 10 seconds.

Use a Pocket Mask

You may give breaths with or without a barrier device, such as a pocket mask. Barrier devices are made of plastic and fit over the person's mouth and nose (Figure 63). They protect the rescuer from blood, vomit, or disease. Your instructor may discuss other types of barrier devices, like face shields, which can be used when giving breaths.

If you're in the workplace, your employer may provide personal protective equipment, including pocket masks or face shields, for use during CPR.

There are many different kinds of pocket masks as well as different sizes for adults, children, and infants. So, make sure you're using the right size. You may need to put a pocket mask together before you use it.

Give Breaths With a Pocket Mask

Follow these steps to give breaths with a pocket mask (Figure 63):

How to Give Breaths With a Pocket Mask
☐ Put the mask over the infant's mouth and nose. • If the mask has a pointed end, put the narrow end of the mask on the bridge of the nose; position the wide end so that it covers the mouth.
☐ Tilt the head and lift the chin while pressing the mask against the infant's face. It is important to make an airtight seal between the infant's face and the mask while you lift the chin to keep the airway open.
☐ Give 2 breaths (blow for 1 second for each). Watch for the chest to begin to rise as you give each breath.
☐ Try not to interrupt compressions for more than 10 seconds.

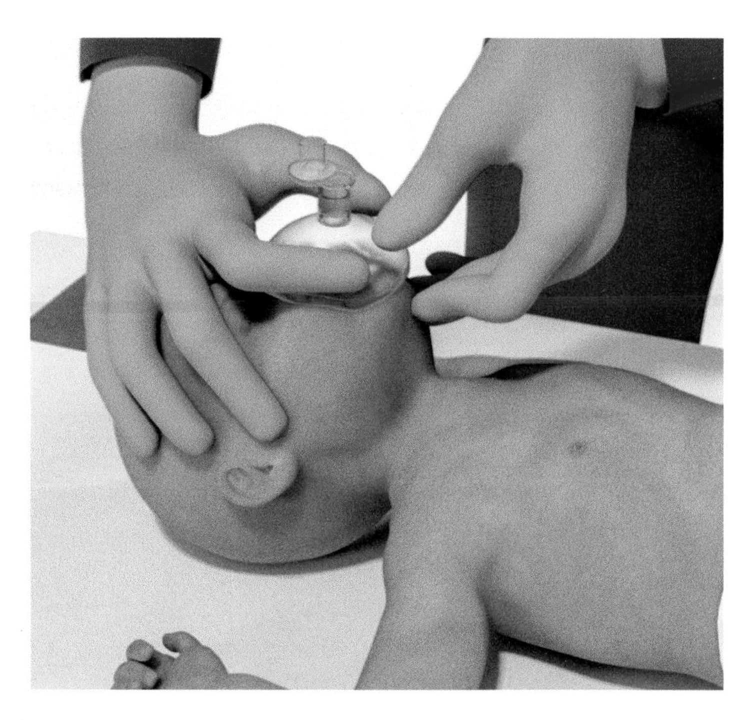

Figure 63. Giving breaths with a pocket mask.

Give Sets of 30 Compressions and 2 Breaths

When providing CPR, give sets of 30 compressions and 2 breaths.

How to Give Sets of Compressions and Breaths to an Infant
☐ Make sure the infant is lying on his back on a firm, flat surface.
☐ Quickly move clothes out of the way.
☐ Give 30 chest compressions. • Use 2 fingers of 1 hand to give compressions. Place them on the breastbone, just below the nipple line. • Push straight down at least one third the depth of the chest or about 1½ inches. • Push at a rate of 100 to 120 compressions per minute. Count the compressions out loud. • Let the chest come back up to its normal position after each compression.
☐ After 30 compressions, give 2 breaths. • Open the airway and give 2 breaths (blow for 1 second for each). Watch for the chest to begin to rise as you give each breath. • Try not to interrupt compressions for more than 10 seconds.

Do Not Delay CPR to Get an AED for an Infant

CPR with both compressions and breaths is the most important thing you can do for an infant in cardiac arrest. Do not delay CPR to get an AED for an infant. If someone brings an AED to you, use it as soon as it arrives. See the "Use an AED" section in "CPR and AED Use for Children."

Putting It All Together: Infant High-Quality CPR Summary

Infants usually have healthy hearts. Often, an infant's heart stops because the infant can't breathe or is having trouble breathing. As a result, it's very important to give breaths as well as compressions to an infant.

Compressions are still very important to deliver blood flow and are the core of CPR. Try not to interrupt chest compressions for more than 10 seconds when you give breaths.

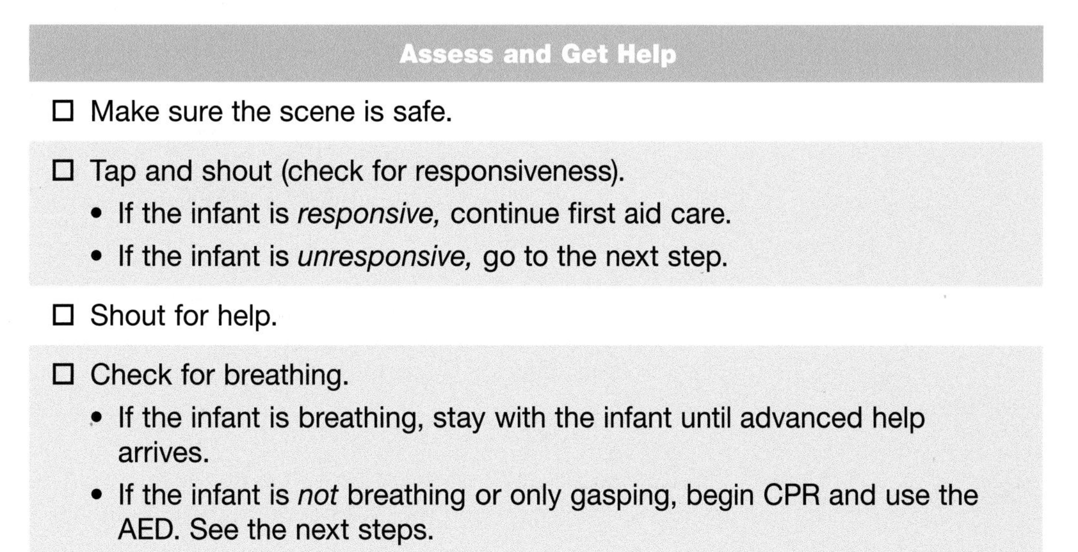

Assess and Get Help

- ☐ Make sure the scene is safe.
- ☐ Tap and shout (check for responsiveness).
  - If the infant is *responsive,* continue first aid care.
  - If the infant is *unresponsive,* go to the next step.
- ☐ Shout for help.
- ☐ Check for breathing.
  - If the infant is breathing, stay with the infant until advanced help arrives.
  - If the infant is *not* breathing or only gasping, begin CPR and use the AED. See the next steps.

Begin CPR, Phone 9-1-1, and Get an AED

- ☐ Begin CPR, phone 9-1-1, and get an AED.

If someone comes to help and a cell phone is available

- Ask the person to phone 9-1-1 on the cell phone, put it on speaker mode, and go get an AED while you begin CPR.

If someone comes to help and a cell phone is not available

- Ask the person to go phone 9-1-1 and get an AED while you begin CPR.

If you are alone and have a cell phone or nearby phone

- Phone 9-1-1 and put the phone on speaker mode while you begin CPR.
- Give 5 sets of 30 compressions and 2 breaths.
- Go get an AED.*
- Return to the infant and continue CPR.

If you are alone and don't have a cell phone

- Give 5 sets of 30 compressions and 2 breaths.
- Then, go phone 9-1-1 and get an AED.*
- Return to the infant and continue CPR.

*If the infant isn't injured and you're alone, after 5 sets of 30 compressions and 2 breaths, you may carry the infant with you to phone 9-1-1 and get an AED.

Provide High-Quality CPR

When providing CPR, you give sets of 30 compressions and 2 breaths.

- ☐ Make sure the infant is lying on his back on a firm, flat surface.
- ☐ Quickly move clothes out of the way.
- ☐ Give 30 chest compressions.
  - Use 2 fingers of 1 hand to give compressions. Place them on the breastbone, just below the nipple line.
  - Push straight down at least one third the depth of the chest or about 1½ inches.
  - Push at a rate of 100 to 120 compressions per minute. Count the compressions out loud.
  - Let the chest come back up to its normal position after each compression.
- ☐ After 30 compressions, give 2 breaths.
  - Open the airway and give 2 breaths (blow for 1 second for each). Watch for the chest to begin to rise as you give each breath.
  - Try not to interrupt compressions for more than 10 seconds.
- ☐ Use an AED as soon as it is available.
  - Turn the AED on and follow the prompts.
  - Attach the pads.
    - Use child pads for an infant if available.
    - If child pads are not available, use adult pads.
  - Let the AED analyze.
  - Make sure no one is touching the infant, and deliver a shock if advised.
- ☐ Provide CPR and use the AED until
  - Someone else arrives who can take turns providing CPR with you
  - The infant begins to move, cry, blink, or otherwise react
  - Someone with more advanced training arrives and takes over

Conclusion

Summary of High-Quality CPR Components

Component	Adults and Adolescents	Children (Age 1 Year to Puberty)	Infants (Age Less Than 1 Year)
Make sure the scene is safe	Make sure the scene is safe for you and the person needing help		
Tap and shout (check for responsiveness)	Check to see if person is responsive or unresponsive If unresponsive, go to next step		
Shout for help			
Check for breathing	If breathing normally, stay with the person until advanced help arrives If *not* breathing normally or only gasping, begin CPR and use an AED	If breathing, stay with the child or infant until advanced help arrives If *not* breathing or only gasping, begin CPR and use the AED	
Begin CPR, phone 9-1-1, and get an AED	Phone or send someone to phone 9-1-1 and get an AED while you begin CPR If you are alone and have a phone, put it on speaker mode and phone 9-1-1 while you begin CPR	Phone or send someone to phone 9-1-1 and get an AED If you are alone and have a phone, put it on speaker mode and phone 9-1-1 while you begin CPR If you are alone and do not have a phone, give 5 sets of 30 compressions and 2 breaths. Then go phone 9-1-1 and get an AED. Return and continue CPR.	
Compressions and breaths	30 compressions to 2 breaths		
Compression rate	Push on the chest at a rate of 100 to 120 compressions per minute		
Compression depth	At least 2 inches	At least one third the depth of the chest, or about 2 inches	At least one third the depth of the chest, or about 1½ inches
Hand placement	2 hands on the lower half of the breastbone	2 hands or 1 hand (optional for very small child) on the lower half of the breastbone	2 fingers in the center of the chest, just below the nipple line
Let the chest come back up	Let the chest come back up to its normal position after each compression		
Interruptions in compressions	Try not to interrupt compressions for more than 10 seconds		

Legal Questions

Good Samaritan laws exist to protect providers who help ill and injured people. The laws vary from state to state. Your instructor will talk to you about the laws that apply to you.

Duty to Provide CPR

Some people may be required to perform CPR while working. Some examples are law enforcement officers, firefighters, flight attendants, lifeguards, and park rangers. If they are off duty, they can choose whether or not to provide CPR.

Providing CPR may be part of your job description. If so, you must help while you're working. However, when you're off duty, you can choose whether to provide CPR.

After the Emergency

If you provide CPR, you may learn private things about a person. You must not share this information with other people. Keep private things private.

Remember to

- Give all information about the person to emergency medical services rescuers or the person's healthcare providers
- Protect the person's privacy

After the Heartsaver Course

Congratulations on completing this course!

Practice your skills. Review the steps in this workbook often. This will keep you prepared to give high-quality CPR whenever it's needed.

It's important to phone 9-1-1 when an emergency arises. The dispatcher will remind you what to do.

Contact the AHA if you want more information on CPR, AEDs, or first aid. You can visit **www.heart.org/cpr** or call 1-877-AHA-4CPR (877-242-4277) to find a class near you.

Even if you don't remember all the steps exactly, it is important for you to try. Any help, even if it isn't perfect, is better than no help at all.

Life Is Why

Science Is Why

Cardiovascular diseases claim more lives than all forms of cancer combined. This unsettling statistic drives the AHA's commitment to bring science to life by advancing resuscitation knowledge and research in new ways.